THE GREAT MENOPAUSE MYTH

THE
GREAT
MENOPAUSE
MYTH

THE TRUTH ON MASTERING
MIDLIFE HORMONAL MAYHEM,
BEATING UNCOMFORTABLE SYMPTOMS
& AGING TO THRIVE

KRISTIN JOHNSON, JD., BCHN FNTP & MARIA CLAPS, FDN-P
DR. CARRIE JONES, TECHNICAL REVIEWER

FAIR WINDS

Quarto.com

First Published in 2024 by Fair Winds Press, an imprint of
The Quarto Group, 100 Cummings Center, Suite 265-D,
Beverly, MA 01915, USA.
T (978) 282-9590 F (978) 283-2742

Fair Winds Press titles are also available at discount for retail, wholesale,
promotional, and bulk purchase. For details, contact the Special Sales Manager by email at specialsales@quarto.com or by mail at The Quarto Group,
Attn: Special Sales Manager, 100 Cummings Center, Suite 265-D, Beverly,
MA 01915, USA.

ISBN: 978-0-7603-8826-6

Digital edition published in 2024
eISBN: 978-0-7603-8827-3

Library of Congress Cataloging-in-Publication Data is available.

Design: Kelley Galbreath
Illustration: Ada Keesler

DISCLAIMER: This book contains our personal and clinical experiences as
well as ideas and opinions we have formed as postmenopausal women working to help other women in this transition. Our intent is to provide helpful
general information on the topics contained herein and is in no way a substi-
tute for the advice of our readers' own medical professionals. Individual help
for any personal symptoms, conditions, or other concerns should be sought
by consulting a skilled and competent physician and/or other qualified
health professional. Many of the recommendations and analyses discussed
in this book are supported by scientific studies and clinical work, and much
of the supporting research is provided in the References section. That said,
together with our publisher, we specifically disclaim all responsibility for any
loss, damage, or injury that someone may incur as a result of following any
advice or suggestions in this book.

To Mom, if only you knew then what we know now, maybe your life would have been better and our relationship could have been different. To Dad, you pushed me to never stop learning and thinking—thank you. I miss you more than words can express.

—KRISSIE

To my husband—the meals you had to cook, the laundry you had to fold, and for my attention you weren't given, all so I could bring this book baby into the world.

—MARIA

CONTENTS

INTRODUCTION

The Great Menopause Myth: How Women
Have Been (Dangerously) Misled About Their Health
and How to Make This Your Best Chapter Yet

THERE IS A WELCOME NEW NARRATIVE for women on midlife, menopause, and aging . . . but it needs a course correction.

Midlife and the menopausal transition are a naturally tumultuous time for women and their health. Disruptions in sleep along with declines in mood, cognition, weight, skin and hair health, and more all get women's attention due to their effect on one's appearance. Up until recently, the messaging around these unwelcome changes in midlife has been that they are an inevitable part of aging and that if women can just white knuckle through the discomfort, it will pass.

Times are changing, however, and now—finally—midlife and menopause are having their moment. Open discussion about midlife and menopause has made its way into pop culture media, showing up in both legacy and alternative outlets, and is the subject of numerous new books on the topic. In addition, the menopause topic is ubiquitous on social media platforms, with loads of speakers, authors, and influencers holding themselves out as "menopause experts." Much of the newer discussion tries to convince women to see menopause as one of two different paradigms. One paradigm is that menopause is a time for empowerment and renewed allegiance to feminism that requires the rejection of the "patriarchy-based" framing of menopause as pathological, a disease process; as a result, this view neglects any interventions that may address menopause. The other paradigm holds that menopause is a time for women to embrace their aging and focus on their innate wisdom while letting their symptoms pass. Regardless of which camp women place themselves in, due to the primary focus of these discussions being on the *visible* signs and symptoms of aging, myriad suggestions offered to help women who choose to take action all have something in common: They are short-term, temporary "fixes" that result in an endless (and ineffective) pursuit of some shiny object that will stop or slow these unwelcome changes.

We agree with both camps that menopause can be an amazing time in a woman's life, and we celebrate and cheer all of the increased awareness around it. Yet, from a health perspective, there is nothing about menopause that makes women healthier. Yes, the global shift in the dialogue around midlife and aging is encouraging, but women are undeservedly being led into the second (and sometimes longest) chapter of their lives focused on the wrong target with the wrong tools. As a result, they remain ill-equipped to avoid the real declines in their health that result from the chronic diseases of aging kicked off by menopause. The reality is that by age sixty, women match or lead men in nearly every disease associated with aging. This is not okay, and it does not have to be an inevitability.

Women don't need more noise—they need agency. We want to help women gain that agency. Rather than being forced to opt into one side or the other of the new menopause narrative, women deserve a deep education about midlife and the myths of menopause so they are fluent in what is happening to their physiology and the drastic changes that will eventually result. With this book, we hope to provide that education.

Everything needs new attention in midlife: nutrition, movement, sleep, stress management, mind-set, gut function, metabolic health, and more. In addition, lifestyle is only half of the puzzle. Understanding hormones, why they are essential, what happens when we lose them, why we've been taught to fear them, and what decisions we can make about them are not topics adequately given their due in the resources currently available. More important, women need this information sooner rather than later so they can start living intentionally in their forties in order to be healthy and thriving in their sixties and beyond—but no one is being open about how time is of the essence. For already postmenopausal women, they need information regarding the options they actually have and how to make decisions that will serve them best. No one is giving women the whole picture, and we are determined to change that.

As postmenopausal women ourselves, we have lived firsthand a variety of partial truths, myths, and downright lies—not just about what was happening to our bodies during midlife and menopause but also about what it meant for our health as well as the options we had to address it. Our respective experiences drove us to pursue additional education, research, and mentorship on the topic of women's hormonal health and the changes known as "menopause." What we learned infuriated—and motivated—us. From research quality being negatively affected due to pharmaceutical interests to treatment options and talking points being predetermined and dictated by medical societies, insurance companies, and regulated licensing agencies, women are being misled about menopause and forced into a single lane for how they age. We believe women deserve to know the truth about this crucial period of life along with all options available to them, and so we have committed ourselves to doing what we can to bring women insight and clarity about their health through our practice, Wise & Well.

For the past ten years, we have been, and continue to be, in the trenches educating and coaching women about midlife and hormonal changes along with effective options they have to protect their health as they age. Even more important, we have been working alongside pioneering medical providers who are committed to changing the standard of care for menopausal women. This has enabled us to dig into these providers' patient data and get an up-close look at the results yielded by the different approaches to treating menopause and its symptoms. Our acquired experience is recognized by medical providers such that we are asked to lecture regularly on midlife women, metabolic health in menopause, and the role of hormone replacement therapy. In addition, we serve on the governing and clinical advisory boards of a nonprofit dedicated to changing the standard of care for menopausal women. As a result, we have both personal and clinical experience that we combine to provide midlife women with specialized and comprehensive education, tools, and focus, tailored to help them positively address the realities ahead.

Although we guide women through the journey of menopause in our private client practice, with this book, we want to provide you the what, why, and how to build a menopause toolbox. We will help you understand the role of nutrition, movement, sleep, stress, and lifestyle on midlife health and why giving them attention is essential for aging in a healthy manner. We will teach you not just what hormones do but also, and more important, what their loss means and the many ways to address the risks that result—whether or not that includes hormone therapy. Our aim is to bring more women the knowledge they need in a comprehensive guidebook with actionable steps from which they can choose their menopause narrative so they may age making informed choices and with their health intact.

PART ONE

HORMONES AND WOMEN'S HEALTH

CHAPTER ONE

MENOPAUSE MYTHS ARE AFFECTING WOMEN'S HEALTH

DID YOU KNOW THAT ONLY 54 PERCENT of women can correctly define menopause? Why and how can a topic so quintessentially female not even be understood by the very group for whom it is solely reserved? The answer lies in the many myths around menopause. Let's explore.

DEFINING MENOPAUSE: MYTHS VS. REALITY

Menopause awareness can be traced all the way back to the ancient Greeks. In fact, the roots of the word *menopause* can be found in the Greek language—*men*, meaning "month," which is related to the word *moon*, and *pauein*, meaning "to cease or stop." Thus, menopause has long been thought simply to be the time when a woman's monthly (lunar) cycle ends. Unfortunately, this description doesn't even come close to the truth.

Due to years of special interest by the medical-industrial complex coupled with various sociopolitical movements, the definition of menopause has become unnecessarily confusing and filled with falsehoods. For example, the push to have patents on hormone therapy has resulted in studies skewed toward less-than-optimal products, thereby negatively affecting the safety data on hormones. Likewise, the rise of a certain variant of feminism has framed the

TRACKING THE
MENOPAUSAL TRANSITION

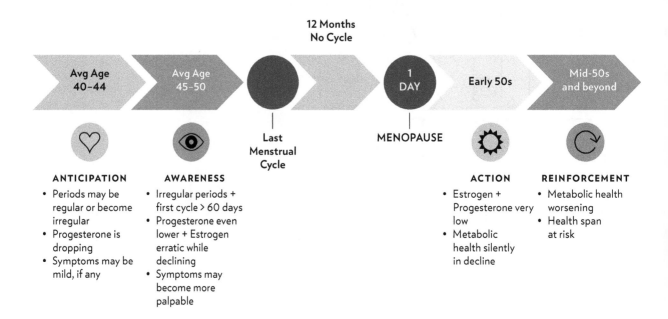

12 Months No Cycle

| Avg Age 40–44 | Avg Age 45–50 | | | 1 DAY | Early 50s | Mid-50s and beyond |

Last Menstrual Cycle

MENOPAUSE

ANTICIPATION
- Periods may be regular or become irregular
- Progesterone is dropping
- Symptoms may be mild, if any

AWARENESS
- Irregular periods + first cycle > 60 days
- Progesterone even lower + Estrogen erratic while declining
- Symptoms may become more palpable

ACTION
- Estrogen + Progesterone very low
- Metabolic health silently in decline

REINFORCEMENT
- Metabolic health worsening
- Health span at risk

use of hormone therapy as an outcropping of patriarchy by maintaining women's appearances. Much of this noise has impacted discussions around hormone replacement therapy (HRT) as an effective means of protecting women's health and, for some women, created "sides" to the issue. Frankly, menopause in its current and modern understanding, is a myth.

- First, we have what **health care providers** tell us from a clinical approach: Menopause is simply the permanent end of menstrual periods and, thus, the end of fertility and reproduction. It is "officially diagnosed" as the date on which a woman has gone twelve months without having a period. Natural menopause is preceded by perimenopause, or the menopausal transition, which can last up to ten years, and the time after the single date of menopause is identified as "postmenopausal." Globally, the average age of a woman at menopause is fifty-one. Menopause can happen significantly earlier, either by surgical removal of a woman's ovaries or by a condition known as "premature ovarian failure," something that has a variety of causes—from genetics to autoimmune processes to cancer therapies and more. In addition, menstrual bleeding can cease with hysterectomy, ablation, or use of an IUD, and women who experience these may not yet be menopausal, making the medical definition useless and confusing. Regardless of cause, the most common symptoms of menopause are hot flashes and night sweats (called vasomotor symptoms, or VMS) but can also include cycle changes and increased vaginal dryness.

- Next, we have what **the media** tells us from a historical approach: Menopause only happens to human females and is relatively new because women used to die much younger and are only now outliving the life spans of their ancestors. Menopause is a normal "hormonal deficiency" that intentionally stops reproduction because if women continued to have babies into old age they would not be around long enough to raise their offspring—and there may be more birth defects due to aging eggs. Menopause is needed so women of this age can help raise grandchildren, thereby helping the human species survive. Menopause should be embraced as a natural, biologically and socially necessary event that liberates women to enjoy sex without fear of pregnancy and that gives them renewed autonomy over their lives and how they choose to live.

- Then, we have what **society** tells us from an ideological approach: Menopause is simply part of aging and women should lean into it. Menopause happens to many more species than just humans and in no way represents a hormonal deficiency because it is nature's planned way of ending reproduction. To speak of menopause as a deficiency is to say that women past menopause are deficient in some way and that their lives have been prolonged past

society's limited intentions for them: reproduction. The concept of hormone deficiency is evidence of bias (induced by the patriarchy) that is ageist and sexist. Women's societal roles extend far beyond just reproduction because their accumulated wisdom is essential for helping their descendants thrive. Menopausal women have exactly the right amount of hormones for this stage of life. Calling it a deficiency is just a commercially motivated perversion to convince women to take HRT.

- Finally, we have what many **women** tell us from a very personal perspective: Menopause is hot flashes, poor sleep, foggy brains, anxious and shifting moods, dry vaginas, fat bellies, wrinkly skin, thinning hair, persistent headaches, leaky bladders, and more! Thankfully, though, when menopause causes these things, medications and lifestyle changes can help women "get through it" while it "passes."

What if we said that ALL these sources of menopause information are getting menopause wrong? (Except the women and their symptoms—there is no denying the lived experience of things women feel and see with menopause!)

Menopause, as a physiologic process, is neither a single moment in time nor does it have an end point. Menopause is not simply about ending fertility and reproduction, regardless of the reason. Menopause is not socially necessary nor should it be deemed desirable and something we need to embrace *or* reject. Menopause is not a liberation for women nor is it a patriarchal, let alone commercial, construct. Menopause is not just about symptoms and uncomfortable changes.

These popular notions of "menopause" are arbitrary and irrelevant constructs that divert attention away from the fact that menopause is really only a tiny part of a larger, longer, and more significant health transition that is occurring—one that *not* telling women about has resulted in millions being denied the opportunity to age healthfully.

Menopause can be both concerning and amazing. Menopause affects multiple systemic processes far beyond fertility and menstruation. Menopause is an acceleration of events that have been occurring long before its natural arrival. Menopause, when premature, is so powerful that it can increase biological age well past chronological age. Menopause is an absence in the body of critical messengers that most physiologic systems rely on to function properly. Menopause is the loss of metabolic balance for women. Menopause is a vital sign—no different than blood pressure or body temperature—that alerts women to disruptions in their bodies shifting them rapidly away from optimal health. Menopause needs your attention.

MENOPAUSE AFFECTS *EVERYONE*

Whether you are a woman or someone who loves a woman, menopause *will* affect you.

Global life expectancy has increased by thirty years since 1950 to approximately seventy-three years old, and yet, despite all the advances of modern medicine and public health initiatives that have helped the world live longer, the quality of women's (extended) lives has not improved. This is what is referred to as the "life span–healthspan gap" or the disconnect between total life lived (life span) and the period of life free from disease (healthspan). Although living longer sounds great, living it disease-free sounds even better. For women, unfortunately, this is not how it works.

In 1900, women's life expectancy was 47.3 years, with the top three leading causes of death being primarily infectious diseases: inflammation of the small intestine and diarrhea, pneumonia and influenza, and tuberculosis. Today, all of those leading causes of women's mortality have been replaced by chronic diseases, specifically cancer, heart disease, and stroke. This shift is indicative of the harsh reality that the additional longevity women have gained since the mid-twentieth century comes with poorer health status.

Although many are quick to chalk up these statistics to aging, in reality, the declines in women's health occur primarily during these relatively new "extra" years, while the same cannot be said for men. In fact, even though men who live to age one hundred are far fewer in number than women who live that long, such men have significantly better physical function and cognition than women of the same age. Additionally, for women who experience menopause prematurely, they, too, suffer from chronic disease at ages much younger than those who experience menopause later. This is not aging—this is menopause.

The data does not lie. Compared with age-matched men over fifty, women tend to have a poorer health status and quality of life:

- **Before the age of fifty,** women are at low risk of developing cardiovascular disease (CVD), but *after* the age of fifty, women's risks increase exponentially as cardiovascular disease becomes the number-one killer of women and puts them on par with men. By age sixty-five, 75 percent of women have high blood pressure, surpass men in the incidence of stroke and aneurysms, and equal men in incidence of heart attack.

- **Women over the age of fifty account for** more than 80 percent of all breast cancer diagnoses and are more likely than men to develop colon polyps, leading to increased colorectal cancer risk.

- **Women over the age of fifty have a four times** higher rate of osteoporosis and a two times higher rate of osteopenia compared to men. These women also represent 80 percent of all osteoporotic fractures and tend to have fractures five to ten years earlier than men.

- **Women over the age of fifty comprise** nearly 70 percent of all clinically diagnosed cases of dementia and Alzheimer's disease—a rate twice that of men.

- **Women over the age of fifty have two to** four times the incidence of anxiety and depression compared to men of the same age.

- **Women over the age of fifty outnumber men** four to one in autoimmune disease diagnoses and up to nine to one with certain systemic autoimmune processes such as lupus.

- **Women over the age of fifty are twice as likely** as men to experience reduced sleep quality as well as increased insomnia and restless leg syndrome compared to men.

It is clear, women may have the advantage when it comes to life span, but they don't have any advantage when it comes to healthspan. This cannot all be reduced down to aging because, while both women and men "age," there is one single health event women experience that men do not: menopause.

Menopause as *just* the loss of fertility and menstrual cycles or the rise of hot flashes and vaginal dryness is a myth. Menopause is a longer life spent with elevated chronic disease and mortality risks. The hard truth is that no woman gets to avoid menopause but she can avoid its impacts, and it is this gap in knowledge that impairs women's health and relationships—significantly.

THE STATISTICS OF MENOPAUSE

By 2030, more than 1.2 billion women worldwide—a full 14 percent of the entire globe and nearly one-third of all women—will be considered postmenopausal. Each year, an additional 47 million women join that statistic. Today, there are 55 million menopausal women in the United States, nearly 75 percent of whom regularly seek support or treatment for physical and emotional changes they attribute to menopause. These changes range from uncomfortable and inconvenient to debilitating and life-altering. Among the most debilitating changes women face are hot flashes, painful sex, urinary tract infections, and the taxing combination of anxiety, brain fog, depression, and insomnia. Given that the average woman will live 40 percent of her life after menopause, it is understandable why women fear it.

Although the symptoms of menopause are significant, so are the mortality implications of menopause. Demographic evidence and clinical studies have long shown that, before menopause, women have a significantly reduced risk of dying from any cause—a term the medical community refers to as *all-cause mortality*. It would be an amazing statistic, if it lasted. The reality is that shortly after the age of fifty, women lose their mortality advantage, and the evidence is clear that this, too, is attributable to menopause. Whether symptoms or disease and death, one thing for certain about menopause is that its effects are difficult to predict and always come at a cost.

A study by the Mayo Clinic published in 2023 was able to put a price on the economic effects of menopause symptoms in the workplace. These costs were defined as those related to the direct and indirect problems of absenteeism, reduced or lost work productivity, increased direct and indirect health care costs, and lost opportunities for career advancement or continued employment. The results are staggering: Lost work time per year costs US employers and employees an estimated $1.8 billion, and $26.6 billion annually when medical expenses are added.

It is not just women, workplaces, and health care that pay the price of menopause. Termed the "gray divorce," marriage problems that occur around menopause currently account for one-quarter of all divorces for women over age fifty. Although the overall divorce rate in the United States has declined, among those age fifty and older, it has roughly doubled since 1990. In the United Kingdom, a survey by The Family Law Menopause Project showed that seven in ten women (73 percent) blamed menopause for the breakdown of their marriage, with 67 percent of respondents claiming it increased domestic abuse and arguments. Although these statistics only demonstrate correlation between menopause and marital breakdown, there are possible explanations for the connection: Menopause negatively alters sexual intimacy with impairment of vaginal tissue and libido; menopause drives mood dysregulation, which intensifies feelings of anger and depression; menopause reduces emotional response, leading to a sense of disconnectedness; and, because men's hormone loss happens much later and more gradually, their empathy and understanding can sometimes be lacking at a time when women desperately need both.

If physical, personal, corporate, and societal costs attributed to menopause are not enough to cause alarm, the statistics on the knowledge gap of our health care system should be. Despite the universality of menopause, medical providers remain ill-equipped to address these issues. According to the United States–based American Association of Retired Persons (AARP), more than 80 percent of graduating internal medicine residents admit they do not feel comfortable, let alone adequately trained, to discuss or treat menopausal women. Even worse, only 20 percent of all residencies in obstetrics and gynecology—a specialty reserved solely for female health—even offer training on menopause.

To us, these statistics are incredibly compelling—and concerning. But more concerning is that, despite these significant issues around menopause, there now exists a market-driven exploitation of women dealing with menopause.

THE MENOPAUSE GOLD RUSH UNLEASHED

While women and their health care providers scramble to figure out how to deal with menopause, private corporations and tech start-ups have wasted no time cashing in on a burgeoning category of products targeting menopausal women. Riding a financial boon referred to as the "menopause gold rush," these companies have brought to market a plethora of wellness products using words like "symptoms," "alleviate," "balance," and "cure" to promote them. Changes in global demographics are on their side, too, and not just because women in menopause make up a large part of the population, but also because women over fifty are increasingly more affluent than ever before. From a market perspective, it is estimated that menopause is a $600 billion opportunity that remains largely untapped. In terms of established menopause products, global sales were $15.4 billion in 2021 and are forecasted to be $24.4 billion by 2030, with dietary supplements leading the growth.

It's not just companies selling products, either. Masking their role as investors in digital platforms offering telemedicine and other services aimed at menopause, celebrities are preying on women's emotions by sharing their personal menopause stories while promoting products marketed as menopause solutions. These marketing tactics have blurred the lines between consumerism and activism. Regardless of the vulnerabilities portrayed by these celebrities, there is no multivitamin, cream, or organic potion that will address the real imperatives of menopause. Given the lack of clarity, education, and effective

health care or other solutions around menopause, however, rather than being consumers, menopausal women have become the product. Caveat emptor.

MAKE SENSE OF IT ALL AND PUT YOURSELF IN CONTROL

We can personally attest that it is a challenge for women to sift through the morass of information about midlife and menopause and find the truth. Women are tired of navigating the sea of confusion, fear, and misinformation around menopause pushed in popular media and, at times, by their own health care providers. After sex education, contraception information, and prenatal classes, women are left to navigate menopause without an accessible compass. It does not have to be this way.

We believe that aging is not about chronological years lived but, rather, about deficiency states in the body, and for women, specifically, that means their sex hormones. If the body is kept in a state of sufficiency rather than deficiency, it has what it needs to work optimally, and this will enable women to delay the arrival of or reduce most of the downstream consequences commonly blamed on aging.

We propose that it is time for women (and society) to reframe the menopause problem: It is not about aging but, rather, as we stated earlier, a vital sign signaling to women that their whole body health is changing. More importantly, menopause is a late signal—sort of like osteoporosis; you usually don't know it is an issue until you have a fracture—and for this reason, women need to learn what is happening with the onset of the menopausal transition, why it matters, and what they can do about it.

Women *can* improve their healthspan and truly enjoy their extended life span. Women *can* make their later years some of their best ever—physically, emotionally, and socially. Women *can* take charge of menopause; all that's needed is a fresh look coupled with sound education that provides them agency to live, and age, healthfully.

Although menopause, hormones, and women's physiology are complex issues, understanding them does not have to be difficult. It all starts with understanding sex hormones and their role in women's whole body health, which we'll explore in chapter 2.

THE MAIN MENOPAUSE MYTHS

Here are just some of the widely believed myths about menopause that we'll dispel in this book. Get ready to change the way you think about menopause!

1 Menopause is simply the loss of menstrual periods and the end of fertility.

2 Menopause is natural and the body will eventually adapt to lower hormone levels.

3 Menopause without symptoms means you have nothing to worry about.

4 Menopause can be adequately managed with the birth control pill.

5 Hormone therapy is only for severe hot flashes and bones that are becoming brittle.

6 Hormone therapy causes cancer and strokes and should be avoided.

7 Testosterone can replace your hormones just fine.

8 A doctor who can prescribe hormone therapy is knowledgeable about it and has your whole body health in mind.

9 There is not much you can do if you can't replace your hormones.

10 Just do what your doctor (or girlfriend) tells you to get through menopause.

CHAPTER TWO

FEMALE HORMONES

Understanding the Changing Midlife Landscape

TO UNDERSTAND WHAT IS HAPPENING to women during the ages of forty to sixty-five or what is otherwise referred to as "midlife," it is important to know some basics about hormones, generally, and sex hormones, specifically. We will also discuss what happens before, during, and after the menopausal transition. We are confident that, with a solid grasp of this information, you will see why maintaining or restoring hormones beyond midlife is so important to women's long-term health.

HORMONE BASICS

Hormones are chemical substances that act like messengers, sent out from our cells to travel through our blood and bodily fluids to tissues and organs. Once they arrive at their destination, hormones deliver a message that affects the functioning of other cells. In simple terms, hormones are important signals our body sends around to different parts of itself. Beyond just the hormones you may know about (such as adrenaline, cortisol, estrogen, insulin, and testosterone), the body actually secretes more than one hundred different hormones. These hormones regulate many physiologic processes throughout the body and influence everything from metabolism to blood pressure, blood sugar regulation, fluid balance, body temperature, growth and development, sexual function, puberty, fertility, reproduction, mood, stress response, sleep, and more.

There are several types of hormones categorized into three distinct groups according to their chemical composition:

1 **Steroids,** derived from fat or lipids

2 **Amines,** derived from a single protein or amino acid

3 **Peptides,** derived from multiple proteins that form a chain

Each hormone group has a different way of traveling and acting in the body due to its individual chemical properties, and although they are all vital and interact with each other, for our purposes, the focus is on **steroid hormones**. The most important thing to know is that hormones are not always present in a constant supply; instead, their production and action are highly dependent on triggers from something called the endocrine system.

The Endocrine System

Each part of a woman's body—from the brain to the skin, heart, kidneys, and muscles—has a specific job to

THE ENDOCRINE ORCHESTRA

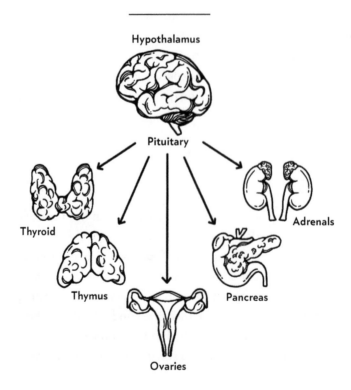

Hypothalamus

Pituitary

Thyroid

Adrenals

Thymus

Pancreas

Ovaries

do. To get that work done correctly, these body parts take instructions from the endocrine system. Made up of a series of glands and other hormone-producing organs, the endocrine system coordinates everything from growth and metabolism to fertility, mood, digestion, and detoxification—and it manages all of this through the production of hormones. We like to describe it as a sort of internal email system: Glands or organs send out hormones to other parts of the body to deliver messages about what work needs to be done, when to do it, and for how long. Think of hormones as "command central" of this internal communication network known as the endocrine system.

The coordinated movement, synthesis (formation), and distribution of hormones within the endocrine system rely on multiple instruments, just like an orchestra. To achieve harmony, all instruments need to play together with precision—if they don't, bodily processes get out of tune and the result is dysfunction. The hypothalamus and pituitary, in the brain, oversee the endocrine system's work. The hypothalamus is a small but mighty part of the brain that sends out hormones that carry *releasing* signals to the pituitary to make it release its hormones. Also located in the brain, the pituitary is considered the master gland, like the orchestra conductor, because it sends out critical hormones that carry *stimulating* messages to the rest of the endocrine system, which, when received, trigger all the jobs to help our body function and stay in tune.

And, although hormones are widely distributed throughout the body and have access to all cells, a given hormone can deliver its signal only to a limited number of cells—those that possess receptors for that specific hormone. These cells are called **target cells**, and a target cell responds *only* to hormones for which it bears **receptors**—a cell protein that is able to receive a specific hormone's signal; thus, cells that do not have such a receptor cannot be influenced directly by that hormone.

An easy way to think about this is to compare it to TV broadcasts. Pretend the endocrine system is a twenty-four-hour television news network. The signal from this network is being broadcast all over, available to anyone within range, BUT only those with receivers tuned to that specific news network's signal will actually get the broadcast.

Hormones and receptors are like that—each hormone has a unique signal that influences only those cells that have receivers tuned specifically for it. The key is that the receiver or receptor must be functioning; if it is not, no signal is received and the important message from the hormone cannot stimulate the action for which it is intended. Hormone receptor function is dependent upon maintaining optimal levels of hormones in the blood and tissues. As important as hormones are, receptors are equally important, because without their action, nothing can be triggered in the body, no matter how important the hormone's message is!

Because there are *many* instruments (glands and tissues) in this incredible orchestra (endocrine system) producing such important sounds (hormones) that then play together to make beautiful music (ensuring proper body function), the body uses a self-regulating process called a *feedback mechanism*, which is a loop in which a hormone feeds back to control its own production. Said differently, **feedback loops** provide the controls needed to keep the effects of hormones and their chain reactions from spiraling out of control.

Feedback loops can be negative or positive.

- In a **negative feedback loop**, hormones are constantly being kept within a particular narrow range despite what is going on around them (like your thermostat maintaining your house's temperature regardless of whether it is hot or cold outside).

- In a **positive feedback loop**, the concentration of a hormone is increasingly intensified until it is no longer needed (such as pressing the gas pedal of your car when passing another vehicle in traffic and then reducing such pressure once safely passed).

Most endocrine hormones are regulated by negative feedback loops, which is important because it means that the endocrine system will bring things back to normal by shutting down manufacturing when levels of output, or the amount of accumulated hormone, get too high. This is called homeostasis, which means the regulation of internal conditions to keep our body functioning at optimal levels, even when challenged by internal and external changes.

For example, feedback loops are commonly referred to as an axis—or a group of glands that signal to each other in sequence—and although we have multiples of these in the body, there are three primary ones that are essential to our health:

1 **HPA:** hypothalamus + pituitary + adrenal, essential for regulating our response to both perceived and physiologic stressors

2 **HPO:** hypothalamus + pituitary + ovaries, essential for the production or inhibition of ovarian sex steroid hormone secretion and function

3 **HPT:** hypothalamus + pituitary + thyroid, essential for thyroid regulation and controlling the synthesis and secretion of thyroid hormones that regulate metabolism and energy expenditure

SCIENTIFIC LITERATURE WILL OFTEN use HPG to denote hypothalamus + pituitary + gonadal axis, where gonads connotes the non-gender-specific sex organs. HPO is used when specifically discussing women, referring to the ovaries.

Continuing this example, using the HPT axis (hypothalamus + pituitary + thyroid), the hypothalamus secretes thyrotropin-*releasing* hormone, or TRH. TRH stimulates the pituitary gland to produce thyroid-*stimulating* hormone, or TSH. TSH, in turn, signals the thyroid gland to secrete its hormones. When the level of thyroid hormones is high enough, the hormones will "feed back" in reverse to stop the hypothalamus from secreting TRH and the pituitary from secreting TSH. Once that TSH stimulus is turned off, the thyroid gland stops secreting its hormones.

This example of a feedback system is quite simplified. In reality, the body relies on very complex positive and negative feedback systems, often involving multiple different hormones and tissues to regulate bodily functions. If the feedback loop is disrupted, or not working, conditions such as *hypo*thyroidism (underfunctioning) or *hyper*thyroidism (overfunctioning) result. Because the thyroid is the primary player in regulating metabolism, people with these conditions will experience symptoms such as, in the hypofunction,

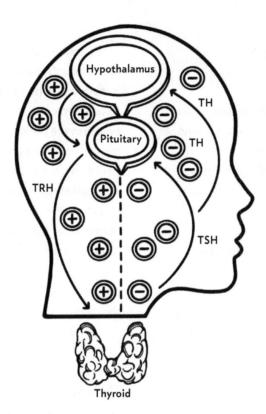

Thyroid

weight gain, fatigue, constipation, depression, weak muscles, or foggy brain, or, in hyperfunction, weight loss, heart palpitations, heat intolerance, irritability, increased sweating, or vision changes.

When disordered function occurs due to a problem with the gland responsible for secreting the hormone, it is considered a primary disruption to the feedback loop. That said, feedback loops can also have disordered function due to secondary disruptions, such as developmental failures, hypothalamic/pituitary problems, receptor issues, nutrient deficiencies, toxin exposure, surgical disruptions, and even stress, whether acute or chronic. Although in today's modern world secondary disruptions are increasingly more common, midlife and women's hormone problems are

due to primary disruption—more on that later.

So, when any one of these hormone feedback loops becomes disordered for any reason—primary or secondary—the entire body's stability, or homeostasis, becomes disrupted, and a variety of problems arises, some of which we may become aware of (via symptoms) and others that we are often unaware of (via disease processes) . . . until it is too late.

And although all hormones and endocrine feedback loops matter for our health, to understand the profound changes that affect women's quality of life and disease risk at midlife and beyond, we need to go a bit deeper and talk specifically about the HPO axis (hypothalamus + pituitary + ovaries), its sex hormones, and ovarian function decline.

SEX HORMONES AND THEIR FEEDBACK LOOP

The HPO axis is activated at puberty and its production and regulation of specific steroid hormones control a woman's sexual development, menstrual cycle, reproductive capacity, and aging. For women, HPO steroid hormones and where they are released are as follows:

- From the hypothalamus → gonadotropin-releasing hormone (GnRH)

- From the pituitary → gonadotropins, specifically luteinizing hormone (LH) and follicle-stimulating hormone (FSH)

- From the ovaries → estrogen, progesterone, and testosterone

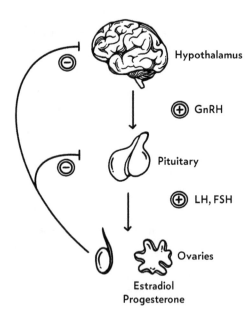

Hypothalamus

⊕ GnRH

Pituitary

⊕ LH, FSH

Ovaries

Estradiol
Progesterone

Estrogen is produced primarily by the ovaries in reliable amounts in the premenopausal years. Progesterone is made *only* when a woman ovulates, and then testosterone is made in the ovaries, adrenal glands, and other tissues in the body. Once produced, these hormones travel throughout the body to their target cells and then bind to sex hormone receptors on the cells, specifically estrogen receptors alpha and beta, androgen receptors, and progesterone receptors. Think of this binding of sex hormones to their receptors as a lock and key, where the receptor is the lock and the hormone is the key. Turning the key sets off a cascade of biological responses inside the cell, helping women's bodies function according to the message or instructions delivered.

Introducing Estrogens

The estrogens are a family of steroid hormones that promote the development and maintenance of a female's body characteristics. Estrogen is made primarily in the ovaries but it can also be produced by fat cells and certain peripheral sites—other parts of the body away from the ovaries. For example, a woman's adrenal glands, stomach, and even brain can each make a bit of estrogen and so are considered peripheral sites.

Although there are many different estrogen-like molecules in plants and animals in nature, a human female makes three major forms of estrogen: estrone, estradiol, and estriol. Each estrogen differs only slightly in structure, but that small difference triggers significantly different actions in our cells.

Estrone, often listed as E1 in scientific literature, has much weaker biological activity than estradiol and binds primarily to estrogen receptor-alpha (ER-α). Although estrone is produced primarily by the ovaries before menopause, it can also be made in fat tissue and the adrenal glands. As women enter midlife and ovarian function declines, estrone becomes the primary estrogen in a woman's body after menopause and is almost entirely from adrenal production and adipose (fat) tissue. It is not well understood what stimulates the production of estrone, but we do know that estrone and estradiol can be converted into each other. Nevertheless, because estrone is weaker than estradiol, it is not considered as important for women's overall health.

Estradiol, listed as E2 in scientific literature, is the main female estrogen throughout most of a woman's life—her premenopausal years. Estradiol is also the most potent of the estrogens and triggers the events necessary for reproduction and whole body health. It binds equally to both estrogen receptors alpha and beta (ER-α and ER-β). Although estradiol is produced primarily within the ovaries, it is also made in significantly smaller amounts in various other tissues, including the brain, breasts, liver, and more. Compared to

A QUICK NOTE ON RECEPTORS

Although hormones are important because of the messages they carry, without adequate healthy receptors to receive them their messages will not be brought into tissues' cells and organs. So, the body's ability to receive and take up hormones is just as critical to overall health as the ability to produce the hormones in the first place.

Estrogen is the only sex hormone with two different subtypes of classic receptors, and they behave quite differently from each other. Estrogen receptor-alpha (ER-α) is responsible for proliferation or growth, whereas estrogen receptor-beta (ER-β) is responsible for stopping that growth. So, think ER-α = accelerator and ER-β = brake.

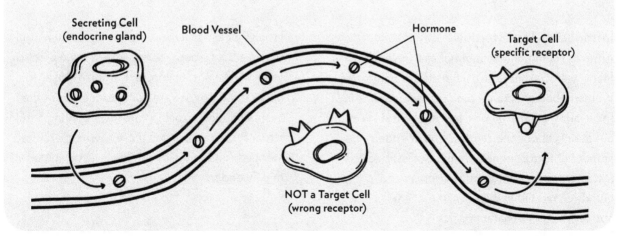

Secreting Cell (endocrine gland) · Blood Vessel · Hormone · Target Cell (specific receptor) · NOT a Target Cell (wrong receptor)

estrone, estradiol has up to five times the potency and up to four times the concentration in a woman's body.

Estriol, listed as E3 in scientific literature, is the main estrogen of pregnancy. Unlike estrone and estradiol, estriol is made not by the ovaries but, rather, is a direct result of estradiol conversion. It is, effectively, a by-product of estradiol, and it binds primarily to estrogen receptor-beta (ER-β). Although it exists in small levels over a woman's lifetime, it is primarily an estrogen of pregnancy and plays no significant role in the health of nonpregnant women.

Introducing Progesterone

Referred to as P4 in scientific literature, progesterone is a natural steroid hormone produced primarily in the ovaries, with a small portion produced by the adrenals. It is released by the corpus luteum and is essential for the menstrual cycle, with its most direct effects being to regulate the lining of the uterus and to maintain pregnancy. In fact, this is where progesterone gets its name: "pro" (supporting) "gest" (gestation or pregnancy).

Introducing Testosterone

Although commonly thought of as a male sex hormone, testosterone is also a female sex hormone. Women's bodies actually produce testosterone in the ovaries, adrenal glands, fat cells, and skin cells but at only about one-tenth to one-twentieth the amount of testosterone as men's bodies. Because testosterone acts differently in women and is quickly converted to estrogen, most females do not develop male characteristics.

SEX HORMONES AND THE MENSTRUAL CYCLE

Now that we've covered the HPO axis, its sex hormones, and their receptors, let's explore their relevance to the female menstrual cycle.

Menstruation is a term used to describe the sequence of events that results in the monthly shedding of a woman's uterus lining. This cycle is driven by interactions between hormones produced by the hypothalamus, pituitary, and ovaries (HPO axis) and runs from the first day of a woman's period up to the first day of the next period. Normal menstrual cycles last, on average, twenty-eight days (but can be anywhere from twenty-one to thirty-five days), with bleeding lasting anywhere from two to seven days. Although every woman's cycle is slightly different, the hormonal fluctuations are the same.

There are two separate but simultaneous cycles that complete menstruation, and they each include different phases—the *ovarian cycle* include the pre-ovulation follicular and post-ovulation luteal phases, whereas the *uterine cycle* includes pre-ovulation, menstruation and

IT MAY SEEM STRANGE to talk about menstruation in a book about menopause, but we promise you it is relevant, no matter a woman's age! To understand why, we are going to talk about the events happening *behind the scenes* during a menstrual cycle because it is these events that, when stopped, lead to the health declines of women in midlife and beyond.

PHASES OF THE MENSTRUAL CYCLE

CYCLE	Pre-ovulation		Ovulation	Post-ovulation
OVARIAN CYCLE	Folicular phase			Luteal phase
UTERINE CYCLE	Menstruation	Proliferative phase		Secretory phase

the proliferative phase, ovulation, and the post-ovulation secretory phase.

Pre-ovulation stimulates actions within both the ovaries and the uterus. This first part of the cycle starts during the few days a woman's levels of estrogen and progesterone are at their lowest. These low levels cause the top layers of the uterus's lining (the endometrium), which has thickened in preparation for a possible pregnancy, to break down and shed, thereby triggering a menstrual bleed. In response to this, the pituitary increases FSH output to stimulate the development of fluid-filled sacs in the ovaries, called follicles, where eggs can mature (also known as the **follicular phase**). From these, one follicle gets selected to become a mature follicle destined to ovulate, called the *dominant follicle*. As the dominant follicle matures, it increases estrogen production, which causes FSH to decrease. As estrogen levels rise, the lining of the uterus begins to grow and thicken gain (also known as the **proliferative phase**).

Ovulation happens when the brain sends a surge of LH and FSH to the ovaries, stimulating the dominant ovarian follicle to rupture and release an egg. During this surge of LH and FSH, estrogen hits a peak level for the menstrual cycle.

Once ovulation occurs and the egg is released, the **luteal phase**, which lasts about fourteen days,

starts and the pituitary responds by decreasing the levels of LH and FSH. This decrease closes the ruptured follicle in the ovary and forms a remnant called the corpus luteum, which produces progesterone in increasing amounts until it peaks about a week into the cycle. During most of this phase, estrogen production remains high and, together with progesterone, causes the endometrial lining of the uterus to thicken more and secrete special proteins in preparation for possible fertilization (the **secretory phase**). If the egg is not fertilized (pregnancy), the corpus luteum breaks down and the production of progesterone starts to decline. In response, estrogen also declines and the top layers of the uterine lining break down and shed, triggering a menstrual bleed and the entire cycle to repeat (see illustration on page 34).

Essentially, what the menstrual cycle represents is a beautiful rhythmic dance between the brain and the ovaries with regular and robust fluctuations in hormones but always a Day 12 estrogen peak followed by a Day 21 progesterone peak. Over a woman's lifetime, this cycle repeats itself every month from puberty until around the early forties, when, as midlife approaches, things start to change with the HPO axis and a woman's production of sex hormones.

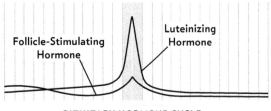

PITUITARY HORMONE CYCLE

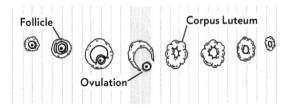

OVARIAN CYCLE

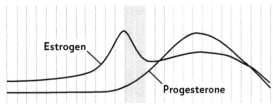

SEX HORMONE CYCLE

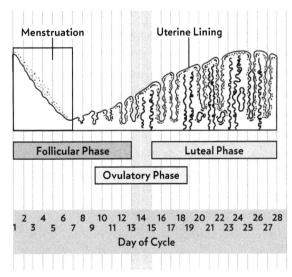

ENDOMETRIAL CYCLE

IN OUR OPINION, one of the great tragedies in the education of women is the lack of information they are given about their menstrual cycle as adolescents, particularly in the United States. Adolescent girls, if anything, are taught to loathe their cycle, believing it to be merely a monthly nuisance they must endure. We promote that this needs to change because, once women understand menstruation, we believe there will be much less celebration around its departure in menopause.

HORMONAL CHANGES IN THE MENOPAUSAL TRANSITION

We've covered some complex information thus far, so if it is new to you, reread it so you feel comfortable with the concepts and terms, but here's a quick recap of the menstrual cycle and the actions of all the players in the HPO axis:

- Start of cycle → estrogen ↓ + progesterone ↓

- Hypothalamus → gonadotropin-releasing hormone ↑ to signal to the pituitary

- Pituitary → follicle-stimulating hormone ↑ to stimulate follicles in the ovaries

- Ovarian follicle → estrogen ↑ so that follicle-stimulating hormone ↓

COMPLETE MENSTRUAL CYCLE

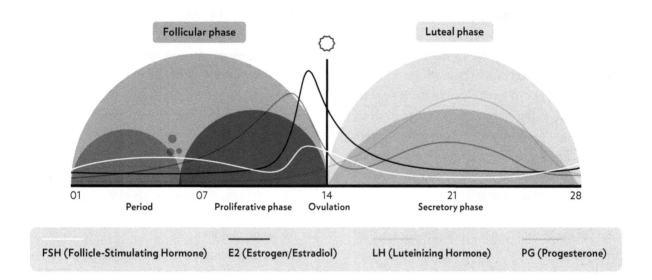

Follicular phase   Luteal phase

01   07   14   21   28

Period   Proliferative phase   Ovulation   Secretory phase

FSH (Follicle-Stimulating Hormone)   E2 (Estrogen/Estradiol)   LH (Luteinizing Hormone)   PG (Progesterone)

- Dominant follicle selected → egg development starts!

- Pituitary → surge of estrogen ↑ and follicle-stimulating hormone ↓

- Peak of estrogen stimulates the egg to mature → surge of luteinizing hormone ↑ and follicle stimulating hormone ↑

- Ovulation → dominant follicle releases an egg → luteinizing hormone ↓ follicle-stimulating hormone ↓

- Follicle becomes corpus luteum → progesterone ↑ to a peak, estrogen stable

- No fertilization/pregnancy → progesterone ↓ and estrogen ↓

Visually, this looks like the image above.

During the fertile years between puberty and the beginning of the menopausal transition, also called perimenopause, this tightly choreographed dance within the HPO axis continues to perform beautifully; eventually, however, the music stops, and not only does that window of fertility close but also a woman's monthly period stops. The question becomes, why?

Got Eggs?

Although it may not be obvious, if we look at this cycle in reverse, from the end to the beginning, the rhythm of the phases and cycles of the HPO loop are highly dependent upon the development and release of an egg, as well as whether said egg becomes fertilized. Here's the problem: Women come out of their mother's womb with a reserve of all of their ovarian eggs—thought to be between one and two million—and are not capable of making new eggs after this. In fact, as women grow, menstruate, and age, there is a continuous decline in the total number of eggs each month. By the time puberty arrives, only about 25 percent of a woman's lifetime total egg supply remains and, over the course of the next thirty to forty years, as the menstrual cycle repeats every month, the entire egg supply gets depleted to zero.

Now, think of ovarian eggs declining to zero in the context of the HPO axis and how the loop of communication might be affected:

- Start of cycle: estrogen and progesterone are at their lowest

- Hypothalamus → gonadotropin-releasing hormone ↑ to signal to the pituitary

- Pituitary → follicle-stimulating hormone ↑ to stimulate follicles in the ovaries

- ~~Ovarian follicles → estrogen ↑ so that follicle-stimulating hormone ↓~~ DOES NOT HAPPEN

- ~~Dominant follicle selected → egg development starts!~~ DOES NOT HAPPEN

- ~~Pituitary → releases a surge of estrogen ↑ and follicle-stimulating hormone ↓~~ DOES NOT HAPPEN

- ~~Peak of estrogen stimulates the egg to mature → surge of luteinizing hormone ↑ and follicle stimulating hormone ↑~~ DOES NOT HAPPEN

- ~~Ovulation → dominant follicle releases an egg → luteinizing hormone ↓ follicle-stimulating hormone ↓~~ DOES NOT HAPPEN

- ~~Follicle becomes corpus luteum → progesterone ↑ to a peak~~ DOES NOT HAPPEN

- No fertilization/pregnancy → progesterone → + estrogen →

As the list shows, the ultimate result of declining follicles eventually reaching zero is high FSH and low estrogen and low progesterone. Visually, this looks like the graph at right.

As the graph on page 37 shows, during perimenopause, the regular and controlled production of FSH, estrogen, and progesterone controlled by the HPO axis starts to falter, creating disorder in the feedback loop. Although the ovaries can still make progesterone, it is at a level significantly lower and lower over time. Likewise, although the ovaries can still make estrogen, it is not reliably in the proper quantity—sometimes too little, sometimes too much, and sometimes just right—while also declining. Finally, FSH continues to increase without any brakes. As a woman's follicle supply winds down and her ovaries head toward full retirement, the ovarian-brain connection of the HPO axis doesn't just falter but disconnects altogether, leaving estrogen and progesterone to bottom out entirely.

No more eggs means no more menstruation and fertility—isn't that a good thing? For a variety of reasons, the short answer is no. Because of its significant connection with fertility, the importance of the HPO axis, its sex hormones, and their receptors is frequently framed as being relevant only during

STAGES OF HORMONES OVER TIME

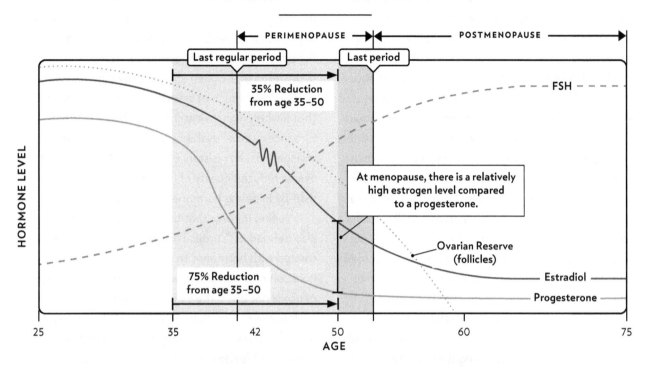

a woman's reproductive lifetime. Remember from chapter 1, clinically, menopause is defined as simply going twelve months without a period, but this view is flawed. Yes, we need to menstruate to be fertile and reproduce, but most women have never been told that there are critical nonfertility-related biological events such as bone remodeling and brain protection (more on these coming up!) entirely dependent on the regular cycles initiated and controlled by the HPO axis and its production of sex hormones. For this reason, the erratic, unpredictable, and eventual halt of ovarian hormone production during perimenopause is incredibly disruptive to women's health.

The menopausal transition is defined as the two to ten years before the final menstrual period when sex hormones are produced both in an unpredictable,

erratic manner and are, ultimately, headed downward. And sometimes, the clearest signals of the onset of this transition are physical symptoms. For some women, this may be irregular and changing menstrual periods, mood changes, hot flashes, weight gain, and disrupted sleep. For others, it may trigger anxiety, brain fog, heart palpitations, vaginal dryness, loss of libido, rising cholesterol, insulin resistance, and more. And while these symptoms absolutely cause discomfort for women who experience them, not all women suffer from noticeable symptoms during the menopausal transition. Just as every woman's menstrual cycle has some variability, so, too, does every woman's transition to menopause.

What is universal for all women, however, is that sex hormones act profoundly to maintain health far beyond the menstrual cycle and so losing them significantly and negatively affects a woman's overall health and disease risk after the transition. In the next chapter we will show you all the actions of sex hormones that are rarely discussed.

It's also important to note that this *isn't* just about aging. If that were the case, then the disappearance of hormones and ensuing disruptions at any age should be of no consequence. Rather, it is well recognized that whenever the body loses its homeostatic adjustment capability (when it loses the function of those important feedback loops we discussed), such loss leads to failure in various adaptive mechanisms, which results in dysfunction, disease, and, ultimately, death. A perfect example of this is the progressively stronger views regarding the menstrual cycle and its connection to women's *overall*—not just reproductive—health.

The National Institutes of Health states that "[t]he menstrual cycle . . . reflects a person's overall health status and can be thought of as a 'fifth vital sign,' along with blood pressure, body temperature, heart rate, and respiratory rate." The American Congress of Obstetricians and Gynecologists enthusiastically shares this view, as do multiple medical journals and physician organizations.

It is clear that having robust and optimal cyclic hormones—as evidenced by the menstrual cycle—is essential for women's good health. Accordingly, any change in a female's period is considered a potentially major warning sign that something, even nonreproduction related, is wrong and, more important, needs attention. In fact, whether a woman wants to have children or not, the absence of a period (amenorrhea) is immediately investigated and usually receives some sort of medical intervention, often including hormone treatments.

Similar to this, when a woman of any age has her ovaries removed (or even damaged due to chemotherapy or other causes), the standard of care is to avoid the adverse health consequences that result from the deprivation of estrogen and other ovarian hormones post-surgery—such as severe vasomotor symptoms (hot flashes, night sweats), mood disorders, sleep disturbances, sexual dysfunction, joint pain, adverse lipid changes, insulin resistance, increased belly fat, and overall reduced quality of life with increased disease risk—by initiating hormone replacement.

We find it ironic that the removal of ovaries is also defined as "surgical menopause" and must be treated with hormones to prevent significant deterioration of a woman's health *and yet* natural menopause is not given the same view or treatment.

It is clear, then, that regardless of the cause, once the ovaries are no longer able to participate in the HPO feedback loop *at any age*, a woman's health starts to decline. So, doesn't it make sense that, rather than viewing low hormones as a result of aging, it is much more logical to consider that "aging" occurs *because of* low hormones?

If menstruation is a critical indicator of women's health far beyond fertility, you are likely wondering what it is, then, that those ovarian hormones are doing outside of assisting reproduction. We're glad you asked—those hormones are doing **so much** and we can't wait to share that with you.

What you're about to learn may make you angry and, ultimately, ask why we are so quick to overlook the loss of hormones when women hit midlife. That's okay, it means you're starting to see the great menopause myth!

CHAPTER THREE

FEMALE HORMONES BEYOND FERTILITY

Effects of Estrogen and Progesterone on Whole Body Health

ALTHOUGH THE VAST MAJORITY OF DOCTORS and women's health professionals have likely told you that your sex hormones are primarily necessary only for fertility and reproduction, those same doctors and health professionals also consider women's periods to be critical vital signs of whole body health at ages before menopause. The presence of a normal menstrual cycle not only signals that a woman is fertile and that pregnancy has not occurred, but also serves as a catalyst for biological events all over the female body: More than four thousand gene products and four hundred physiologic processes in a woman's body depend on *estradiol* and *progesterone*. More important, it is not just the presence of these hormones in the body but also their fluctuations, specifically their cyclic rhythmic dance that includes those peaks we talked about in chapter 2 (peaks of estradiol on Day 12 and progesterone on Day 21), that are essential for triggering cellular behavior that keeps women's bodies healthy.

When women lose their cycle for any reason before the age of 40, conventional medicine warns that the loss of sex hormones results in multiple health risks, including menopausal symptoms such as hot flashes, decreased bone density and increased risk of fractures, early progression of cardiovascular disease, psychological effects that may include depression and anxiety, early decline in cognition, and dry eye syndrome. The widely accepted medical solution is to immediately begin replacing and restoring sex hormones to premenopausal levels to decrease health risks and increase quality of life for these women. So, if sex hormones triggering a proper menstrual cycle are essential for women's health before menopause, aren't the actions of those same sex hormones critical to a woman's health no matter her age or whether her uterus is still intact? Once you learn more about these actions, we are confident you will agree that the answer is clearly yes.

In this chapter and the next, we are going to go through the body, part by part, and demonstrate the most compelling ways that estradiol and progesterone act far beyond fertility. Keep an open mind and be ready to unlearn much of what you have been told about sex hormones and women's whole body health. You will soon realize that women's health has been portrayed wrongly for too long.

MITOCHONDRIA: THE POWERHOUSE YOU DIDN'T KNOW YOU DEPEND ON

Mitochondria are miniature organs, called *organelles*, inside our cells that serve as powerhouses, or energy factories, and are vital to our survival. The energy generated by mitochondria provides the necessary, optimal fuel for our metabolism, or all the chemical processes going on continuously inside our bodies that allow life and normal functioning (homeostasis). This important energy production role means mitochondria are present in nearly every cell we have, with the actual number depending on each type of cell's energy needs. For example, liver cells have more than two thousand mitochondria whereas mature red blood cells have none.

Mitochondria, Apoptosis, and Health

Although mitochondria get the most attention for being energy generators and controlling metabolism, they actually have many jobs, with one of the most important being *apoptosis*. Apoptosis, also referred to as selective or programmed cell death, is what we like to compare to cleaning up messes and taking out the trash to maintain our home's environment. The body's cells are constantly going through life and death cycles and apoptosis is the process by which deteriorating cells are regularly turned over and cleaned out to make room for new, healthy cells. Without apoptosis, dysfunctional and dead cells would pile up, which is akin to letting expired food sit in your fridge, never throwing it out. The result would be loss of homeostasis leading to degeneration and disease. For this reason, mitochondrial control of apoptosis oversees the pace of cells' life cycles and clears out what is not needed, ensuring our bodies are constantly maintained. Accordingly, any impairment in mitochondrial function means our bodies start to decline. Although some people blame mitochondrial dysfunction on aging, we can support mitochondrial function if we support that which influences it—hormones.

Mitochondria and sex hormones have a special love affair. For example, estradiol, progesterone, and testosterone direct mitochondrial actions in every cell of the body, especially in the nervous system and skeletal muscles. Likewise, mitochondria play an essential role in the generation of estradiol and progesterone in a woman's ovaries, adrenals, and brain. Additionally, estradiol regulates mitochondrial energy production by transporting and converting glucose as needed. Estradiol is also required for the regulation of an enzyme called superoxide dismutase, which is needed to detoxify the waste products that are a normal by-product of mitochondrial energy burning. Finally, estradiol determines the protein content and activity of mitochondria as well as the way mitochondria use nutrients to keep their membranes healthy and energy production robust. For their part, mitochondria store calcium, which is crucial for directing the signals of estradiol, progesterone, and testosterone. If anything, mitochondria are dependent on sex hormones for optimal function!

ESTRADIOL AND PROGESTERONE are essential for mitochondrial function.

BRAIN, MOOD, AND SLEEP

It goes without saying that the human brain is our most important organ, serving as command central for our nervous system and controlling our thoughts, memory, movement, and emotions. Obviously, then, maintaining a healthy brain throughout our life span is, hands down, the primary goal in pursuing health and longevity as we age. As essential as the brain is, very little recognition is given to its relationship to our sex hormones.

Estradiol's impact on the brain starts in utero on a developing fetus and continues throughout a woman's life. Estradiol increases the number of progesterone receptors in the brain and progesterone complements the impact of estradiol on the brain; when in ample amounts, they work together to influence higher brain functions such as balance, cognition, emotions, fine motor skills, learning, memory, mood, and motivation. Estradiol also has anti-inflammatory and antioxidant properties that stimulate and regenerate nerve cells to help protect the brain against neurological damage as well as neuropsychiatric conditions—from bipolar disorder to Alzheimer's disease. Finally, estradiol helps mood by modulating pain pathways as well as by influencing the systems controlling our mood chemicals (neurotransmitters) serotonin, dopamine, and norepinephrine.

The brain is one of the primary places in the body where progesterone, like estradiol, has equally broad effects. Not only are progesterone receptors found on most brain cells but also every type of nerve cell contains progesterone receptors. For this reason, progesterone supports brain function by acting specifically on the nervous system through regulation of nerve cell production and regrowth as well as formation of the protective sheath around nerves, which allows their signals to travel quickly and efficiently (called nerve myelination). Progesterone and its downstream products (called metabolites) also influence emotional processing, mood, and cognition by interacting with GABA, the brain chemical that creates calm and eases anxiety. Finally, progesterone suppresses brain swelling, stabilizes brain mitochondria, limits the death of healthy brain cells, and helps correct and maintain homeostasis after brain injury.

ESTRADIOL AND PROGESTERONE are brain protective.

BONES AND SKELETAL STRUCTURE

To remain strong, our bones undergo a continuous remodeling process whereby mature bone tissue is removed and new bone tissue is formed; this not only maintains the body's skeletal structural integrity, affecting posture and mobility, but also contributes metabolically to the body's critical balance of the minerals calcium and phosphorus. Specialized cells in bones—osteoblasts, osteocytes, and osteoclasts—all have estradiol receptors. Estradiol directly acts on these cells to promote building and decrease breakdown of bones, making it the key regulator of bone remodeling cells.

In addition, as part of bone remodeling, osteoclasts must undergo apoptosis, which estradiol also promotes. For bones to heal from injury, they depend on special proteins connected to the immune system. Estradiol controls the balance of these proteins to favor bone building. Estradiol also promotes the production of healthy synovial fluid, which reduces inflammation in joints.

Bones are also affected by special cells of the immune system called T cells. When these immune cells proliferate or multiply, bone can be lost quickly. Estradiol controls the number of T cells to ensure a controlled immune response in favor of supporting bone.

ESTRADIOL is bone protective.

EYES, EARS, AND MOUTH

Our eyes are protected by a three-layer tear solution made up of two types of glands in the eyelids. Via our tear ducts, the layers created by these glands provide important lubrication and protect the eyes not only from drying out but also from being vulnerable to bacteria, microbes, and irritants. Just beyond these outer layers are the cornea and retina of the eye, both of which we are entirely dependent upon to help our eyes focus light so we can see objects near and far clearly. Estradiol and testosterone receptors are found lining not only the glands that provide the outer layers but also along the cornea and retina.

Hearing is one of our most important senses, enabling us to connect with the world around us, maintain family and social relationships, participate in activities, and fully experience life. How we hear is an impressive and complex sequence of steps involving our outer ear, eardrum, tubes, canals, nerves, and hairs, all of which contain important cells responsible for carrying various signals that, ultimately, get translated by our brain into sounds we recognize and understand. Every part of our hearing architecture contains both ER-α and ER-β as well as secondary estrogen-related receptors that play important roles in modulating the signaling involved in hearing as well as protecting our hearing physiology and maintenance, particularly by regulating proper blood flow and circulation to these structures.

Although not as well appreciated as our eyes and ears, oral health is also an important part of and has a direct effect on whole body health, playing a critical role in not only speech and sound production but also serving as the first step in digestion and as a means of breathing and respiration. Multiple structures consisting of both soft and hard tissues with different functions make up the oral cavity, and each is sensitive to changes in the oral environment. Surprising to many, our salivary glands, oral mucosa (the membrane lining the mouth), and periodontal tissues that surround and support our teeth and jaw bones are covered in estrogen receptors, with estrogen serving to maintain saliva levels, keep tissues moist, and regulate bacterial levels in the mouth.

ESTRADIOL is protective of the eyes, ears, and mouth.

SKIN, HAIR, AND MUCOSAL BARRIERS

Our skin is the body's largest organ and comes into contact with our physical world more than anything else. Skin holds in body fluids, prevents us from becoming dehydrated, and keeps out microbes and bacteria that could threaten our health. In addition, our skin is full of nerve endings that help us feel things like heat, cold, and pain. Finally, our skin is an organ of detoxification and its condition plays a huge role in our physical appearance and self-image. Our skin is lined with both estradiol receptors, ER-α and ER-β, which act in all types of cells and layers of our skin. Via these receptors, estradiol acts to protect the appearance and function of skin by maintaining its hydration, elasticity, and thickness and also plays a supportive role in wound healing. This relationship is not one-way, as our skin actually acts as an endocrine organ, producing and releasing estradiol and utilizing enzymes to convert estrogen precursors.

Ask most any woman about her hair, and she will tell you how important it is to her self-image and appearance. Hair is simply a fiber made up of dead cells and consists of two parts—the hair follicle and the hair shaft. The hair follicle has a life cycle that is divided into four distinct phases: anagen (growing phase), catagen (transition phase), telogen (resting phase), and exogen (shedding phase). The hair cycle, as well as the structure of the hair follicle, are highly affected by various hormones. In terms of estradiol and progesterone, their receptors can be found throughout follicles and the scalp and influence the telogen-anagen transition. Estradiol and progesterone, accordingly, have a stimulatory effect on hair growth by shortening the resting phase and prolonging the hair growth phase. In doing so, they not only help our hair stay on our heads longer but also help it grow faster.

The entire *inside* of our body, along the eyes, nose, mouth, throat, sinuses, lungs, gut, and urinary and reproductive tracts, is lined by a thin membrane called the mucosa. The mucosa acts like the skin on the outside of the body, forming a barrier between the bloodstream and everything we inhale and ingest from the outside world. All these mucosal barriers play an integral role in our health by providing structural defense, hosting the microbiome, and housing 80 percent of the body's immune cells. Even with its broad presence throughout the body, our mucosa is extensively lined with estrogen receptors and its health is uniquely dependent upon estradiol. Estradiol regulates the strength of the junctions of this membrane, manages the protective flora contained on and in it, and influences its susceptibility to inflammation, thereby strengthening its defensive actions on our whole body health.

ESTRADIOL is protective of skin, hair, and mucosa.

WEIGHT AND METABOLISM

Metabolic health is highly dependent on balanced blood sugar, low levels of belly fat, healthy cholesterol and other lipids, and proper inflammation control. Although it is often thought that metabolism—the chemical (metabolic) processes that take place as our body converts what we eat into energy—and weight are affected primarily by what and how much we eat and exercise, in reality, our sex hormones have a significant impact on these things.

Estradiol and progesterone both have powerful effects on fat by dictating how much fat we store and where we lay it down. Although progesterone tends to stimulate hunger, both estradiol and progesterone speed up the rate at which we burn calories (our metabolic rate). Estradiol also plays a crucial role in keeping blood sugar stable, particularly by improving how we use glucose and keep insulin levels in check (called insulin sensitivity). Lower insulin, in turn, keeps hunger in check and can accelerate our metabolic rate and stimulate greater fat burning (called lipolysis). Estradiol also supports the production of a hormone called adiponectin, which is essential for the body to lose weight via fat loss. Finally, estradiol prevents atrophy of smooth muscles that can result from high blood sugar.

ESTRADIOL AND PROGESTERONE are metabolically protective.

LIBIDO AND ORGASM

Sex drive depends on a multitude of factors, is very complicated, and is highly individual. Things such as stress, time constraints, conflict, caregiving, mood, and physical pain all play a role in our desire for sex and the outcome we can expect when engaging in sex. Nevertheless, it is well known that hormones profoundly affect a woman's sex drive and, by extension, the ability to have an orgasm. While (sometimes too) much credit is given to testosterone's role when it comes to libido, it is estradiol that profoundly affects female sexual functioning by acting on the central nervous system to create and increase sexual desire. In addition, estradiol is responsible for maintaining the elasticity and flexibility of vaginal tissues, or vaginal tone, as well as increasing vaginal lubrication, all of which determine the comfort of vaginal penetration, arousal, and a woman's ability to climax.

ESTRADIOL is protective of sexual function.

MUSCLES AND CONNECTIVE TISSUES

Muscles attached to bones for movement and strength are called skeletal muscle and, similar to bones, they are constantly undergoing a form of remodeling, or producing new muscle tissue in a process called muscle protein synthesis. Skeletal muscle also has precursor cells, called "satellite cells," that continuously expand, differentiate, and renew themselves to preserve muscle regeneration.

Different from skeletal muscle is smooth muscle, which makes up most of the soft structures of the body's insides, such as the intestines, digestive tract, uterus, bladder, lungs, reproductive organs, eyes, and other areas. The health and integrity of blood vessels within and feeding into these smooth muscle structures are crucial to their (and our) health. All muscles are vulnerable to free radicals, which, when excessive (called oxidative stress), can damage muscle cell membranes and degrade both mass and strength.

Finally, tendons and ligaments are the tissues that connect bones to each other as well as muscles to bones, and they require proper formation of a special protein called collagen to retain their strength and resiliency. Some find it surprising that all of these tissues also have an interdependency on our sex hormones.

Estradiol receptors exist in all muscle cells and regulates and enhances muscle protein synthesis, thereby increasing and maintaining skeletal muscle mass and strength throughout life. Estradiol at premenopausal levels regulates the process of satellite and muscle cell regeneration; it protects against the loss of fast-twitch muscles that provide power, and limits excessive changes to slow-twitch muscles needed for posture and sustained movement. Estradiol receptors line the smooth muscle tissues throughout the body, including the vessel walls, helping bring in nitric oxide to feed all of the body's soft tissues. Estradiol acts as an antioxidant to limit oxidative damage, stabilize muscle cell

membranes, regulate repair and regeneration, and maintain mass and strength. Estradiol increases the collagen content of tendons and ligaments, protecting their strength while decreasing their stiffness.

ESTRADIOL is muscle protective.

HEART AND VASCULAR HEALTH

The cardiovascular system comprises the heart and the vascular system that circulates blood throughout the body. Damage to this system happens in various ways, but three of the most common causes are decreased contraction strength and relaxation of heart muscles (congestive heart failure), stiffening and narrowing of blood vessels, which triggers high blood pressure and can lead to heart attacks and strokes, and deterioration of blood vessel walls and muscle injury due to high amounts of unstable—free radical—molecules and inflammatory proteins (atherosclerosis).

Crucial to overall health, proper function of the heart and vascular system is surprisingly very much dependent on sex hormones. Estradiol has anti-inflammatory and antioxidant effects that protect against muscle injury due to heart attack. Estradiol also regulates the production and function of smooth muscle cells in the heart, thereby preventing their decline. Estradiol stimulates production of nitric oxide, a molecule required for smooth muscle relaxation that then prevents unwanted vascular constriction and maintains appropriate dilation of blood vessels, enabling blood, nutrients, and oxygen to travel to every part of the body, including the brain, effectively and efficiently. Although estradiol is well studied as a means to lower blood pressure, progesterone also appears to lower blood pressure. Finally, estradiol improves cholesterol and lipid profiles, increases receptors for LDL cholesterol, and reduces the buildup of plaque in our arteries.

ESTRADIOL AND PROGESTERONE are cardioprotective.

BLADDER, COLON, AND MORE

The urinary tract consists of the kidneys, bladder, ureters (tubes of muscle connecting the kidneys to the bladder), and urethra (the tube at the bottom of the bladder leading to the exit from our body). Urination is critical to remove waste products and extra fluids from the body, and for it to occur properly, all parts of the urinary tract need to work together *and* in the correct order. The urinary tract is divided into two parts: the upper urinary tract (the kidneys and ureters) and the lower urinary tract (the bladder and urethra), and it is dysfunction in the lower urinary tract that significantly affects a woman's quality of life. Estrogen is known to have an important role in the lower urinary tract's function by maintaining the strength of the pelvic muscles supporting the bladder (the pelvic floor) as well as the thickness of the urethra, allowing proper pressure, flow rate, and emptying of the bladder. In addition, estradiol and progesterone receptors have been found in the vagina, urethra, bladder, and pelvic floor musculature and play key roles in regulating bacterial species diversity and quantity, modulating inflammatory response, and maintaining tissue health.

Although not a body part frequently discussed, colon health is essential to whole body health. The colon, also known as the large bowel or large intestine, is a large tube whose walls are made up of layers of muscles and tissues; its lining consists of a mucosal membrane, blood vessels, nerve endings, and various glands. These structures act as part of the digestive system, allowing us to recycle, convert, and excrete fuels left over after being used by the body. All of the structural and functional elements of the colon are lined with estrogen receptors, and estradiol acts to maintain the health and integrity of these tissues by regulating cellular signaling in the colon, controlling the relationship between microbes in the colon and the rest of the body, and modulating inflammatory responses by the tissues of the colon.

ESTRADIOL is bladder and colon protective.

MICROBIOME AND GUT HEALTH

The gut microbiome, the collection of all microbes, such as bacteria, fungi, viruses, and their genes, that live naturally on and inside the human body and throughout the gastrointestinal tract, plays a critical role in our health. The gut microbiome has a major and direct influence on metabolism, body weight, immune system function, mood, and appetite. These microbes live mostly in the colon (the lower intestine) and out-number all other cells in the body put together. Because of its intimate contact with the larger immune system, the gut microbiome and any imbalances caused by a lack of diversity therein, called dysbiosis, have a significant influence on modulating the body's health.

Female sex hormone levels, particularly of estradiol, influence the composition of all microbes throughout the body, but especially in the gut. In fact, an estradiol–gut microbiome axis exists with a two-way relationship that involves "cross talk" between estradiol and the gastrointestinal tract. For example, the gut microbiome is one of the principal regulators of how much estradiol circulates in the female body, and sufficient estradiol levels form and maintain the lining of the gut and keep it healthy, elastic, and unaffected by the contents of the gut. In addition, new advances in studying the microbiome have suggested that estradiol and the gut microbiome may act cooperatively to lower the risk of obesity and diabetes. Finally, a subset of the gut microbiome is the *estrobolome*, which comprises the totality of intestinal bacteria needed to process estradiol and lower a women's risk of developing estrogen related symptoms like heavy periods and PMS as well as estrogen-related cancers.

THE ESTROBOLOME

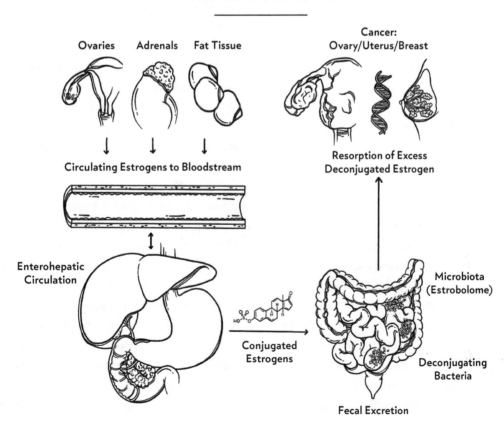

Ovaries   Adrenals   Fat Tissue

Circulating Estrogens to Bloodstream

Enterohepatic Circulation

Conjugated Estrogens

Cancer: Ovary/Uterus/Breast

Resorption of Excess Deconjugated Estrogen

Microbiota (Estrobolome)

Deconjugating Bacteria

Fecal Excretion

Estradiol is also incredibly protective of gut health in that it plays a crucial role in the homeostasis of colon cells. Estradiol also prevents the loss of and promotes the growth of beneficial bacteria that ensure we have healthy diversity in our microbes. Additionally, estradiol decreases the amounts of bacteria, which, when abundant, can trigger inflammation that would otherwise impair the lining of the gut, cross into the rest of the body, and produce a strong immune response. Finally, the fluctuations of estradiol and progesterone in the various phases of the menstrual cycle play an important role in determining how the gut muscles contract and respond to "keep things moving" (called "transit time"), thereby preventing any backup of toxins that could make us ill.

ESTRADIOL is gut protective.

IMMUNE SYSTEM AND ITS BALANCE

The body's immune system is a complex system of organs, white blood cells, antibodies, and chemicals that work together to protect us from foreign invaders such as bacteria, viruses, parasites, and fungi to provide a defense against disease and pathogens. It also takes control of internal homeostasis (clearing debris and repairing DNA damage) and guarantees the recognition of molecules that are either native to the body (self) or foreign (non-self). Although having an immune system able to respond when needed is important, it is equally important that the immune system not overreact and attack cells that are our own—malfunctioning in this way is called *autoimmunity*—and, so, maintaining healthy, balanced function is the key to a strong immune system.

In terms of the immune system's relationship to sex hormones, every type of immune cell is responsive to estradiol and most of them also have progesterone receptors, showing, once again, an important dependency on our sex hormones. For example, estradiol helps support the production of dendritic cells (specialized white blood cells) during inflammatory responses to fight disease and also enhances antibody production (called B cells) to improve virus response. Additionally, estradiol regulates the production and maturation of immune cells, enhancing both our innate rapid immune response as well as our acquired and longer-lasting immune response. In terms of disease protection, estradiol suppresses a particularly pro-inflammatory protein called interleukin-6, which, when left unchecked, can expose us to certain cancers as well as bone and liver diseases.

Indirectly, estradiol helps the immune system by stimulating the production of hyaluronic acid, which protects oral and nasal passageways from viruses, and also increases nasal secretions that contain special molecules with antibacterial and antiviral properties (such as mucus and other immune system proteins), which help combat upper-respiratory infections.

Progesterone also plays a role in our immune response. Progesterone blocks pro-inflammatory immune proteins while stimulating anti-inflammatory proteins. Additionally, progesterone can enhance T cells that protect the body from infection and may help fight cancer. Progesterone also helps remove organisms (pathogens) that produce disease in the body by enabling the destruction of special white blood cells (called natural killer, or NK, cells) that engulf and destroy infected and diseased cells, including cancer cells. Finally, progesterone works to increase the positive effects of estradiol on lung tissue by increasing production of special growth factors that promote lung repair.

ESTRADIOL AND PROGESTERONE are immune protective.

YOUR BREASTS AND CANCER RISK

As previously discussed, every cell in the body has a life cycle in which its DNA is constantly being surveilled so it can be retained, repaired, or passed along. If there is an error in this system that interferes with the normal replication and replacement of cells in the body, mistakes or mutations remain uncorrected, leading to loss of stability in the cell cycle, with the ultimate result being cancer growth. Whether we like to think about it or not, everyone has cancer cells in their body, but the immune system keeps these cells under control by managing cellular life cycles. One player in this management system is a special gene called p53, nicknamed the guardian of the genome, which acts as a primary tumor suppressor and plays a crucial role in maintaining control over the cell cycle's proper function: promoting growth arrest, DNA repair, and eventual apoptosis, the regulated death of the cell when it is damaged beyond repair. Sex hormones play an important role in the actions of the p53 gene. In fact, it is the distinct rhythm and peaks of estradiol and progesterone over the twenty-eight days of the

female menstrual cycle that specifically bring about this p53 suppressor gene's actions.

Beyond regulating the p53 tumor suppressor gene's actions, women's sex hormones have also been shown to be protective against specific cancers. For example, both high and low levels of estradiol and progesterone in pregnancy protect against breast cancer. Additionally, estradiol and progesterone act as protectors in the proliferation and apoptosis of colon cancer cells. Estradiol exposure has also been shown to reduce the risk of gastric cancer, whereas progesterone has been shown to protect against endometrial cancer.

Sex hormones, particularly estradiol and progesterone, have a broad and compelling influence on the female body far beyond fertility. Nevertheless, it is not just the presence of these hormones but, rather, their rhythm (progesterone cycling), amplitude (Day 12 estradiol peak and Day 21 progesterone peak), and physiologic levels (those of a healthy young woman) that are essential. At the onset of the menopausal transition, the period known as perimenopause, these sex hormones begin a descent out of physiologic levels and lose their rhythmic cycling and robust peaks. Because of their influence throughout the female body, unbeknownst to most women, this loss of robust levels and rhythmic cycling has profound effects on women's health, whether symptoms are seen or felt. In the next chapter, we explore what that involves.

ESTRADIOL AND PROGESTERONE are cancer protective.

CHAPTER FOUR

MIDLIFE CHANGES

Why Women Need to Take Charge Before the Signs and Symptoms Start

MANY WOMEN WONDER WHY THEY SHOULD BE CONCERNED with declining sex hormones, often asking, isn't it normal? We respond by pointing out that there are multiple hormones in the body that, when below healthy physiologic (normal) levels, are considered to present as a disease or medical condition deserving treatment. So, why are sex hormones any different? For example, growth hormone deficiency in children is treated by giving human growth hormones; thyroid hormone deficiency is treated by giving thyroid hormones; insulin production problems, such as with diabetes, are treated by giving insulin; low cortisol or aldosterone production, such as with Addison's disease, are treated with corticosteroid hormones. In other words, there are multiple hormone deficiency states for which it is the standard of care to provide medical treatment that involves replacing and restoring the specific hormone to optimal physiologic levels . . . and yet similarly replacing sex hormones in women is *not* the standard of care.

As we made clear previously, estradiol and progesterone act physiologically to maintain the health and normal functioning of many aspects of women's bodies—far beyond fertility and reproduction. As a consequence, it should be expected that the loss of these hormones, for any reason, will play a significant role in the development of diseases, resulting in symptoms, decline, and, ultimately, loss of function.

We concede that, sure, aging is normal, but losing one's quality of life is far from optimal and, frankly, should not be acceptable. Nevertheless, conventional medicine continues to refuse to recognize that these physiologic levels of sex hormones are essential to a woman's healthspan and see no reason to replace them (although some exceptions will be made for debilitating hot flashes or advanced osteoporosis, but not always), despite the fact that they routinely replace thyroid, insulin, growth hormones, and more.

And yet, with women, modern medicine frequently does not even consider replacing women's estradiol and progesterone to improve and maintain healthspan. We want you to understand the consequences of this as well as why you need to pay attention sooner rather than later.

SYMPTOMS ARE PRECURSORS TO LOSS OF FUNCTION AND DISEASE

Instead of looking at menopause as if it is simply the end of fertility and menstruation, we want you to think about the feedback loops you learned about earlier, particularly ovarian function. As we lose follicles, our ovaries slow down and eventually shut down. This is known as *senescence* and, essentially, means that cells are losing their ability to divide and maintain any life/death cycle, which includes sex hormone production. Because we have sex hormone receptors throughout almost all tissues in our body, as this ovarian senescence happens, it translates

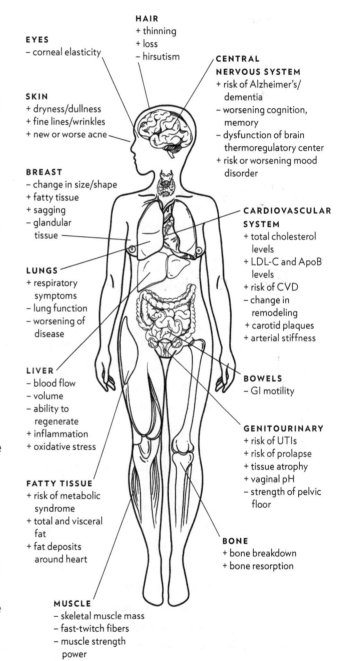

MENOPAUSAL CHANGES

HAIR
+ thinning
+ loss
– hirsutism

EYES
– corneal elasticity

CENTRAL NERVOUS SYSTEM
+ risk of Alzheimer's/ dementia
– worsening cognition, memory
– dysfunction of brain thermoregulatory center
+ risk or worsening mood disorder

SKIN
+ dryness/dullness
+ fine lines/wrinkles
+ new or worse acne

BREAST
– change in size/shape
+ fatty tissue
+ sagging
– glandular tissue

CARDIOVASCULAR SYSTEM
+ total cholesterol levels
+ LDL-C and ApoB levels
+ risk of CVD
– change in remodeling
+ carotid plaques
+ arterial stiffness

LUNGS
+ respiratory symptoms
– lung function
– worsening of disease

LIVER
– blood flow
– volume
– ability to regenerate
+ inflammation
+ oxidative stress

BOWELS
– GI motility

GENITOURINARY
+ risk of UTIs
+ risk of prolapse
+ tissue atrophy
+ vaginal pH
– strength of pelvic floor

FATTY TISSUE
+ risk of metabolic syndrome
+ total and visceral fat
+ fat deposits around heart

BONE
+ bone breakdown
+ bone resorption

MUSCLE
– skeletal muscle mass
– fast-twitch fibers
– muscle strength power

51

into disruption to and senescence of cells and tissues in other areas of the body as well. Here is a visual example: Does this look like simply the end of having babies or does it look like more is at stake?

You may be wondering, if all this is true, why are we not more aware of it? Part of the answer is that, often, much of this happens *slowly*. In fact, it is part of a long progression that starts with symptoms, some of which may be noticeable, others very subtle, that, over time, turn into functional losses, which often end in disease.

For example, when progesterone drops off and estradiol starts its erratic decline, many women in midlife experience brain fog, with things like forgetfulness, lack of focus and mental clarity, even confusion. Oftentimes, we dismiss issues like these to lack of sleep or being stressed but, over time, this brain fog starts to translate into functional declines. This decline in physical and/or cognitive functioning occurs when a person is unable to successfully engage in activities of daily living, such as losing the ability to multitask and manage complex projects, which often impacts job performance, volunteer work, and even meeting the needs of our families. Ultimately, as functional declines persist and advance, the greater concern is that, left unaddressed, this hormonally driven cognitive decline turns into dementia or Alzheimer's disease. Because these changes happen over this sort of "arc of aging," not much attention is given to it, and by the time we have any disease process, it is accepted as normal.

We find it infuriating that no one's really connecting the dots from disease development back to those early symptoms and perimenopause due to sex hormone loss. To give you an idea of how "global"

the effects of ovarian senescence and menopause are on a woman's body, we are going to look at many of the same things we discussed in chapter 3, but this time through the lens of low hormones.

WELCOME TO THE STATE OF INFLAMMATION

One key function of estrogen is its work as a powerful agent in controlling and reducing inflammation in the body. When estrogen levels become erratic and lose their rhythmic cycles, certain immune responses are activated body-wide, particularly in our innate or inborn immune system and its *inflammasome*. The inflammasome is a system of receptors made up of a complex network of proteins that drive inflammatory responses in the body. When these receptors are repeatedly and chronically activated due to low sex hormones, the result is a persistent state of low-grade inflammation. In fact, this inflammasome complex has been found in the cerebrospinal fluid of postmenopausal women, demonstrating how profoundly impactful low hormones are on the body and health of women. Left unaddressed, chronic inflammation (slow, long-lasting inflammation present for prolonged periods) damages healthy cells, tissues, and organs—and the hormone receptors on them—causing changes in the DNA of once-healthy cells. Ultimately, because inflammation plays a central role in the development of various diseases, systemic inflammation driven by low hormones that result from ovarian senescence is a threat to women's quality of life and leaves them susceptible to significant disease risk.

Not surprisingly, when initiated early on in the menopausal transition, *properly** replacing a woman's sex hormones has been repeatedly shown to reduce systemic inflammation, thereby lowering the risk of chronic disease as women age.

* **WE ARE GOING TO HOLD BACK** on the nuances of hormone replacement until later in this book. For now, we want you to know that not all hormone replacement is equal and, when studies show negative effects from hormones, it is often due to the forms and regimens tested. At all times we are referencing **proper** forms, which will be presented to you in detail.

MITCHONDRI*WHAT?*

As a refresher, mitochondria are essential for our health, not only as energy production factories but also as overseers of the maintenance, survival, life cycle, and well-being of our cells. More importantly, mitochondria and a woman's sex hormones, estradiol in particular, have a two-way love affair that is key for homeostasis in the body. When estradiol starts its decline in the beginning of the menopausal transition, it directly impairs mitochondrial function, resulting in disruption of mitochondrial homeostasis, decreased energy flow to the brain and skeletal muscles, increased stress on antioxidant defenses in the body, and lowered whole brain function. Since mitochondria play an essential role in the generation

of sex hormones, their dysfunction disrupts stable production of estradiol and progesterone as well. Essentially, the loss of ovarian hormones precipitates a decline in mitochondrial function that turns into a vicious loop that drives impairment of whole body health and, in particular, brain health, in women.

IMPORTANTLY, STUDIES HAVE SHOWN that replacing estrogen can prevent the harmful effects of cognitive aging and decreases the risks of dementia, provided it is initiated early.

FOGGY BRAIN, ANXIETY, DEPRESSION, AND SLEEP LOSS

Although the menopausal transition is traditionally viewed through the lens of the changes in the reproductive system, the symptoms of this transition largely involve the brain and central nervous system. The reason for this is that multiple estradiol-regulated systems, including those that maintain body temperature (thermoregulation), sleep and our response to light and dark over twenty-four hours, and our sense of the environment around us (sensory processing), are disrupted as hormones decline, and this affects our brain's function. Specifically, the estrogen receptor network becomes uncoupled from our energy systems, which leads to hot flashes, depression, and subjective and objective memory deficits. It is not just estradiol loss that affects brain function, however, as progesterone plays a key role in brain energy, and its drastic reduction is very palpable for women.

Although we are not exactly aware of the internal effects on brain function, we are often acutely aware of how it plays out. For women approaching menopause, one of the most common complaints is foggy brain, whereby they experience difficulty remembering tasks and see a decline in the ability to multitask. This gradual decrease in memory is such a slow decline that, over time, women can unknowingly progress to senile dementia. Studies have shown that midlife women's brains have higher tau, a protein associated with various brain diseases including Alzheimer's, compared with the brains of age-matched men. The earlier a woman experiences menopause, the more elevated the tau.

After foggy brains, poor sleep—whether delayed onset or middle of the night disruption—is the second biggest problem during the menopausal transition. Additionally, women whose hormones are declining are at a two- to fourfold increased risk for massive mood shifts, including new or worsened anxiety and clinical depression, reduced emotional processing, and apathy. Finally, the brain effects of the menopausal transition often result in lower cognition, generally, with declines in memory as well as lower verbal test scores affecting both vocabulary and comprehension.

LOGICALLY, STUDIES SHOW THAT, on balance, proper hormone replacement improves low mood and cognitive changes that occur due to low hormones; however, these effects appear to be most beneficial when hormone replacement starts early in the menopausal transition.

CREPEY SKIN, THINNING HAIR, RINGING EARS, DRY EYES, BURNING MOUTH, AND MORE

It is universally accepted—although a bit begrudgingly so for some—that our outward appearance changes with age. Regardless of one's position on whether presenting a youthful appearance is important, the truth is that some parts of our aesthetics are relevant indicators of our underlying health. For example, skin may develop wrinkles as we age, but whether that skin is also still able to provide an adequate buffer to bruising or heal from cuts and wounds is what matters. Likewise, our eyes may lose some lashes or be less plump as we age, but a marker of their health is more about whether they maintain lubrication and can focus appropriately. The menopausal transition is a time during which many women become aware of significant changes to their outward appearance, regardless of the healthy habits they may have maintained up to that point, and the issues with this go far beyond standards of beauty.

Skin aging is the result of a combination of chronological, environmental, genetic, and hormonal factors. Many women, however, detect a swift acceleration of skin aging symptoms upon entering the menopausal transition. One of the first symptoms noted is an increase in skin dryness, followed by decreased firmness and elasticity. Studies show that the progressive decline in skin thickness is due mostly to the loss of dermal skin collagen and reduced rates of collagen deposition. What these studies also show is that collagen levels in skin directly correlate to estrogen levels. In other words, estradiol deficiency accelerates the loss of skin elasticity by triggering structural changes in elastin fibers due to this loss of collagen, leading to wrinkle formation. Even women who have their ovaries removed before menopause report skin that is thinner and more prone to wrinkles, showing that it is estrogen loss, not aging, that changes women's skin. When skin loses its structure, it becomes itchy and fragile and can bruise more easily, break open, and bleed. Likewise, estrogen-deficient skin is less able to sense touch, pressure, vibration, heat, and cold, leaving women vulnerable to injury.

THANKFULLY, REPLACING ESTRADIOL has been shown to be both protective against and restorative for aging skin in women who have reduced skin health due to estrogen loss.

Regardless of one's position on "looking older," few women would ever admit to having no issues with hair loss as they age. Unfortunately, hair loss is quite common during and after the menopausal transition, affecting more than 40 percent of women. Because of estradiol's and progesterone's protective effects on hair health and life cycle, when these hormones drop, hair follicles start to shrink and hair grows more slowly and becomes much thinner. In two-thirds of women,

this will be all over the scalp, but for the remainder, the hair loss is over the front or temples only.

FOR WOMEN WHO CHOOSE TO replace estradiol and progesterone, however, this hair loss can be halted and hair growth and health can be restored.

Although not fully understood, it is believed that because of the protective role estradiol plays on hearing via its influence on estrogen receptors in ear cells and auditory pathways, low estradiol levels can result in hearing loss for women in midlife and beyond. Hearing loss is more than just an obstacle to communication, and its negative effects permeate and influence all aspects of the lives of those afflicted. Age-related hearing loss is a natural process that occurs as ear structures gradually degenerate with age, but the menopausal transition actually exacerbates this by further reducing blood flow to the cochlea. This change in blood flow harms the sensitive hairlike structures in the inner ear that send sound signals to the brain for interpretation, further worsening women's hearing loss. Additionally, the changes in circulation leave midlife women particularly at risk for developing tinnitus, or ringing in the ears.

WHEN ESTRADIOL LEVELS ARE RESTORED to premenopausal levels, however, hearing sensitivity and regulation are significantly improved.

More than just a nuisance, dry eyes can pose significant problems for women's health. During the menopausal transition, more than 61 percent of women are affected by dry eyes. Lower levels of both estradiol and progesterone cause glands in the eyes to produce less of the oil and fluids necessary for and protective of eye health. This increased dryness can lead to eye allergies, itching and burning, excessive tearing, grittiness, and blurred vision. Worse, however, is that when eye health is impaired due to fluid loss, the eyes become susceptible to the autoimmune disease Sjögren's syndrome, the main symptoms of which are dry mouth and dry eyes.

ALTHOUGH FEW STUDIES EXIST showing a clear consensus of the effects of replacing hormones on dry eyes, estradiol added to eye drops has been shown to improve menopausal women's eye health and function significantly.

A lesser known and somewhat peculiar issue that some women experience in the menopausal transition is a condition called burning mouth syndrome (BMS). When this strikes, women have a burning or scalding sensation in the mouth that can affect the gums, tongue, lips, inside of the cheeks, roof of the mouth, and sometimes even all these areas at once. Burning mouth syndrome can come and go, or persist constantly, and may even trigger a change in the senses of taste and smell. Although the exact causes of BMS are not well understood, statistically, it affects women at much higher rates than men and most frequently

occurs during or after the menopausal transition. Likewise, reduced salivation and changes in the composition of saliva that are common during the menopausal years can significantly affect the health of a woman's oral tissues, teeth, and periodontium as well as increase susceptibility to infections and mechanical injuries. Researchers believe these oral changes are likely related to drops in both estradiol and progesterone, which implicates the importance of the sex hormone receptors that line the mouth and their role in regulating saliva levels and preserving the moistness of tissues and membranes inside the mouth.

ALTHOUGH STUDIES EXAMINING the role of replacing sex hormones and the impact of such on burning mouth syndrome (BMS) are conflicting, these studies did show that women who use hormone replacement therapy have fewer incidences of BMS *and* that when women's hormones are restored, the flow of unstimulated saliva was universally increased, boosting overall oral health.

Given that the inner skinlike barrier or mucosa covers nearly our entire body, damage to its integrity has detrimental effects on our health. When this barrier is broken down, it becomes more permeable than it is supposed to be, which makes it easier for harmful particles, including allergens, bacteria, molds, viruses, and more, to get inside the areas these barriers are meant to protect. When those things get into the body, they trigger the immune system inappropriately and, ultimately, cause inflammation. This inflammation further damages our mucosal barrier and leads to a host of modern diseases such as autoimmune conditions, allergies, bloating, depression, anxiety, digestive issues, mental fog, sleep disturbances, weight gain, and more.

THANKFULLY, VARIOUS STUDIES looking at the mucosa in different areas of the body have shown beneficial effects of proper estradiol replacement to stimulate estradiol receptors for maintaining the membrane's health and permeability.

BLOOD SUGAR CONTROL AND BELLY FAT

One of the most common complaints of women going through the menopausal transition is that, despite a consistent nutrition and exercise regimen, their body starts to change in ways they do not feel they can stop. Whether it is weight gain (an average of 1.5 pounds [680 g] per year) or simply changes in the shape of one's body, this can be very upsetting to midlife women. Even for women whose scale stays the same, weight tends to shift from the butt and hips to the belly area. Making matters worse, women's bodies in midlife tend to get "softer" due to loss of muscle tissue that accompanies this stage of life. Alongside these changes in body mass and shape, midlife women also experience a change in their blood sugar regulation by unknowingly losing sensitivity to insulin, which then drives up cravings, energy problems, and diabetes risk.

The impact of estrogen's loss on metabolic changes in midlife women cannot be overstated, particularly its unique relationship with insulin. Insulin is a hormone produced by the beta cells of the pancreas, and its primary job is to help blood sugar (glucose) enter the body's cells to be used for energy. Additionally, insulin acts as an anabolic or storage hormone by depositing glucose and proteins into muscle tissue and signaling the liver to store glucose for later use, often in the form of fat. Estradiol works to control the rate at which insulin works by applying the brakes on its storage actions and, in doing so, protects us from accumulating fat. Estradiol also directs the location of insulin's storage action by directing it away from the belly.

When a woman's sex hormones drop in midlife, she loses those various control mechanisms on insulin, which results in huge changes in energy metabolism (usage of fuels) as well as disorders with cholesterol and triglycerides (lipid abnormalities in the blood). Over time, what midlife women experience are a lower metabolic rate, depletion of muscle mass, increased belly and visceral fat (fat deposited deeply around our organs, including the heart), and poor blood sugar management. Dysregulated insulin combined with estradiol loss drives midlife women's bodies toward insulin resistance and metabolic disease, which also increases our cardiovascular disease risk.

MULTIPLE STUDIES HAVE SHOWN that replacing sex hormones provides protection against the development of insulin resistance and its negative health consequences.

DOES YOUR LIBIDO NEED A SEARCH-AND-RESCUE TEAM?

Women's sex drive, also called libido, is without a doubt very complex and multifactorial, and for no two women is it the same. Nevertheless, an incredibly common complaint by women is that both their sexual desire and their arousal seem to take a dramatic drop, if not disappear entirely, in midlife and beyond. Without a doubt, the basket of life's burdens in our forties, fifties, and sixties—taking care of kids, partners, parents, and careers—can drive exhaustion and stress that then play a role in our sex drive going on hiatus. But what's really at play is the loss of sex hormones during this same period. Although a belief exists that testosterone is essential for libido, this is neither supported by the studies on women's libido nor does it line up with the hormonal realities of menopause. Whether natural or surgical, menopause's primary influence is on sharply dropping estradiol and progesterone, not testosterone (which declines much more slowly, and later, thanks to continued production via the adrenal glands), and it is the loss of these hormones that is ultimately responsible for a woman's libido going missing.

There are two mechanisms by which estradiol affects sexual drive and arousal. First, estradiol influences libido by acting directly on the central nervous system (our brain!) by keeping our interest in and physical response to sex high. When estradiol is low, these things are blunted. Indirectly, depression and low mood also have a significant impact on libido, arousal, and orgasm, and low estradiol and progesterone are both widely accepted as making midlife women vulnerable to mood changes. Second, sex drive, arousal, and orgasm have a significant physical aspect in that they are dependent upon appropriate responses in a woman's vaginal tissues. When estradiol and progesterone drop, vaginal tissues become dry and thin and lose their flexibility. Additionally, glands in these tissues are responsible for lubrication, which reduces friction and increases pleasure. When sex hormones are low, women lose this natural lubrication, leading to significant discomfort with any penetration. Finally, we need good blood flow to the vaginal tissues to enable them to plump up and lengthen so as to achieve orgasm, but drops in estradiol change blood flow such that we lose our ability to coordinate our brain and body's response to sexual activity.

ALTHOUGH SOME WOMEN INSIST that testosterone replacement has restored their sex drive, unfortunately, the levels of testosterone needed to have this effect are at "supraphysiological" levels, meaning amounts significantly higher than what is normal or ever found naturally in a woman's body.

THANKFULLY, IT IS WIDELY ACCEPTED that when estradiol is replaced in the body to levels similar to those that existed before the menopausal transition, libido can be restored for a satisfying sex life as women age!

FROZEN SHOULDERS, TENDONITIS, ACHY JOINTS, AND HOLE-Y BONES

Sex hormones play a key role in the structure, function, and collagen composition of most connective tissues and joints throughout the body. Estrogen plays a significant role in stimulating bone growth, reducing inflammation and pain, and promoting connective tissue integrity. Loss of estradiol impairs not only the vascular system feeding these structures, but also their strength, flexibility, and range of motion. Specifically, low estradiol contributes to cartilage degeneration, which results in bones rubbing together, causing stiffness and the development of bone spurs, all of which trigger a vicious cycle of further stiffness, pain, swelling, and inflammation that ultimately affects the surrounding tendons and ligaments. As tissue health decreases, midlife women are left with swelling and pain that not only impairs their mobility and quality of life but also leaves them vulnerable to injuries and loss of mobility. In fact, frozen shoulder (adhesive capsulitis) is a condition that predominantly and commonly affects women between the ages of forty and sixty—in other words, women in the throes of hormone loss.

Protecting connective tissue and joint health is essential for preserving women's quality of life during and after the menopausal transition.

Osteoporosis is a "silent" disease that develops when bone mineral density and bone mass decrease. Typically, women do not have symptoms of osteoporosis, and may not even know they have the disease until they break a bone. Osteoporosis is the major cause of fractures in postmenopausal women. Osteoporosis starts about ten years before menopause, when estrogen begins its progressive decline. Bone loss accelerates dramatically during late perimenopause and continues through early postmenopause, resulting in loss of more than 10 percent of bone mass in the first five years after menopause. Estradiol prevents cellular senescence and bone loss: When estradiol is low, the rate at which bones break down is greater than the rate at which bone tissue is formed, creating a net result of osteoporosis, leaving women at incredible risk of loss of their bone matrix, which can lead to multiple fractures. For more than eighty years, it has been known that estradiol deficiency plays the primary role in driving osteoporosis, but progesterone is also helpful for bone loss as estrogen's partner in protecting bone mineral density.

STUDIES HAVE SHOWN that replacing lost hormones provides sustained protection against joint pain and tissue loss and that not using hormone therapy places women at higher risk for tissue and joint disorders.

REPLACING BOTH ESTRADIOL and progesterone has been conclusively shown to restore proper bone turnover and preserve bone mineral density, more effectively than trials of calcitonin, diphosphonates, fluoride, vitamin D, and high calcium intake.

CHOLESTEROL, PLAQUE, STROKE, AND YOUR HEART

Before menopause, women are at low risk of developing cardiovascular disease (CVD) but after menopause, their risk increases *exponentially* as CVD becomes the number-one killer, putting women on par with men for both incidence and severity. In fact, CVD is presently the leading cause of death for both women and men, accounting for one in every three deaths in the United States, and over eighteen million deaths globally. The decline and loss of estradiol affects smooth muscles throughout the body and, as it pertains to the heart and blood vessels, the result is a loss of structural integrity as well as a balanced constriction/relaxation response, which translates into high blood pressure, chest pains, inflammation, and damaged heart muscle. Low estradiol also down-regulates nitric oxide, which is cardioprotective and essential for maintaining the health of our vascular lining. In addition to this, as shown earlier, the menopausal transition increases women's risk of insulin resistance, which significantly affects our CVD risk.

Separate from the direct effects on the heart itself, estradiol also acts protectively on how our body manages cholesterol and other blood lipids. With low levels of estradiol, HDL (good) cholesterol decreases, LDL cholesterol rises, and total lipids in the blood start to increase and modify into unhealthy forms. In addition, the lining of blood vessels becomes damaged and loses vascular tone, which leads to hot flashes and high blood pressure and makes it more likely for plaque and blood clots to form. Finally, there is an increase in fibrinogen, a protein found in blood plasma, leaving women more vulnerable to heart disease, clotting, and stroke.

LOOSE MUSCLES AND LEAKY LADY PARTS

It is undisputed that aging alone can drive losses in muscle mass and strength, but estrogen receptors are present in all musculoskeletal tissues, and estrogen acts directly in these tissues to maintain muscle strength and mass as well as regulate metabolism and whole body health. For this reason, the menopausal transition, and its acute changes in estradiol's availability and effectiveness, actually accelerates and amplifies the negative effects on muscle normally blamed on aging. It is this reality that diminishes the health of midlife women drastically via muscle changes.

From a biomechanical aspect (movement, strength, power, endurance, and function), loss of estradiol results in a decrease in women's ability to produce new muscle (muscle protein synthesis, or MPS), a reduction in their ability to repair muscles and recover after exercise, and a loss of muscle architecture. This means there is a shift from "fast twitch"

REPLACING DECLINING SEX HORMONES has been shown to be a primary preventive therapy for CVD that simultaneously reduces all-cause mortality as well as other aging-related diseases, but its effects are time dependent and best initiated early in the menopausal transition.

(type II) fibers to more "slow twitch" (type I) muscle fibers and a change to shorter and thinner fibers overall, which leads to impairments in walking speed, climbing stairs, balance, and strength. These changes in muscle biomechanical qualities at any age raise women's risk of disability and death exponentially.

Unbeknownst to many is that muscle also has an important biochemical aspect: It plays a vital role in whole body metabolic health. When estradiol is low, women lose their primary reservoir for glucose (blood sugar) storage, which directly elevates their risk of insulin resistance. Additionally, loss of estradiol impairs a woman's ability to dispose of fatty acids (lipids), leading to an accumulation of fat around her organs (visceral fat), increases inflammation by reducing the amount of anti-inflammatory proteins normally released from muscle, and lowers the immune system's strength by altering the activity of mitochondria and detox enzymes in muscle tissue—all of which combine to increase oxidative stress and lower metabolic health in midlife women's bodies. Finally, the interaction of estradiol and muscle directly affects our rate of bone turnover, and the loss of estradiol's influence on muscle in this process leads to further risk to bones.

REPLACING ESTRADIOL HAS BEEN SHOWN to help offset aging-related losses in muscle mass, strength, and function, prolonging women's ability to maintain an independent life; however, these benefits were strongest when estradiol was added earlier in the menopausal transition.

One aspect of the combination of muscle-plus-estradiol loss that is often overlooked is the impact it has on women's bladder control. Muscles create the "floor" of a woman's pelvis and secure the stability and position of the bladder and lower urinary tract. Estrogen and progesterone receptors have been found in the vagina, urethra, bladder, and pelvic floor musculature, and via these receptors, sex hormones act to not only maintain the strength and supportive function of the pelvic floor muscles but also to maintain vascular flow and proper bacterial populations in the surrounding tissues. When estradiol is lost in the menopausal transition, women can develop laxity and atrophy in their pelvic floor, which leads to urinary incontinence and the embarrassing leakage of urine after sneezing, coughing, laughing, or straining, if not total loss of bladder control. In addition, low estrogen means the loss of tissue moistness and protective bacteria in the urinary tract, leaving women vulnerable to burning, itching, pain, inflammation, and urinary tract infections (UTIs).

ESTRADIOL THERAPY HAS BEEN SHOWN to improve tissue health, microbial diversity, and muscle function in the pelvic floor and urinary tract, alleviating the risk of incontinence and UTIs.

BAD BUGS AND GUT PROBLEMS

The gut and its microbiome have a profound impact on our health. Proper functioning of the gastrointestinal (GI) tract and its community of microorganisms helps optimize digestion and bowel movements, destroy harmful bacteria, and control the immune system. Additionally, the gut has an important two-way relationship with estradiol that maintains its health and function via estradiol receptors found throughout the stomach and intestines.

The loss of estradiol in the menopausal transition and subsequent alteration of gut function and the microbiome play a significant role in driving poor bowel health and increased weight gain often seen in midlife women. In fact, a decrease in estradiol and its receptors contributes to the progression of a number of GI diseases, including gastroesophageal reflux (GERD), esophageal cancer, peptic ulcers, gastric cancer, inflammatory bowel disease, and irritable bowel syndrome as well as other gut-modulated diseases such as colon and breast cancer.

When the gut microbiome's health is impaired, it changes the secretion of beta-glucuronidase, an enzyme critically important for the excretion of estrogen metabolites (inactive forms of estrogen left over after the body uses estrogen). When this enzyme's function is impaired, these metabolites can be converted back into active forms of estrogen that get recirculated and absorbed into the bloodstream. This reactivation of previously used and metabolized estrogens leaves us at risk of irritability and mood swings, weight struggles, acne, bloating, and poor digestion. Additionally, because the largest density of immune cells in the body is in the small intestine, when the gut microbiome is impaired due to loss of estradiol, or for any reason, women are more susceptible to food allergies and intolerances as well as seasonal and environmental allergies.

REPLACING LOST HORMONES has been shown to reverse negative gut microbiome alterations, improving gut bacterial diversity, increasing digestion and bowel transit time, reducing recirculation of previously used estrogens, balancing immune response, and mitigating overall disease risk.

HASHIMOTO'S, RHEUMATOID ARTHRITIS, MULTIPLE SCLEROSIS, AND OTHER AUTOIMMUNE PROCESSES

When our body's natural defense system cannot tell the difference between our own cells and foreign cells, the body can mistakenly attack normal cells. This is called an autoimmune process and can affect a wide range of body parts. Autoimmune diseases presently affect millions of people, but women far outpace men in terms of diagnosis rates as well as constitute more than 85 percent of individuals with multiple autoimmune diseases worldwide.

Autoimmune disease is highly influenced by inflammation, and many studies suggest that the menopausal transition exerts a profound effect on autoimmune risk via estrogen deficiency–driven changes in the immune system. Specifically, midlife women's immune systems can experience deterioration in the function of the thymus, the primary organ of the immune system, as well as changes in the function of white blood cells that protect us from infection (T cells and B cells), stable production of antibodies, and general immune response and tolerance. Additionally, a low estradiol state predisposes women to higher rates of new autoimmune disorders and worsening of the symptoms of autoimmune diseases acquired before the menopausal transition.

IN NEARLY ALL TYPES of autoimmune disease, replacing estradiol has been shown to improve symptoms and disease progression.

CANCER, BOOBS, AND BIRTHDAYS

Ask any woman about one of her biggest fears as she ages and she will undoubtedly mention cancer, particularly breast cancer. Sadly, the vast majority of physicians have been (wrongly) taught that hormones "cause" cancer, and so most women now believe the same. The flaws in this belief system are based largely on poorly designed and interpreted studies (about which we will have plenty to say later), but they are also a result of confusing "controlling" with "causing." As we have (hopefully) shown in this and the previous chapter, hormones are incredibly powerful and have significant positive influences on our health as women. In fact, if they posed a real risk to women's health, then none of us who have borne children would have survived pregnancy (when our hormone levels are at peak highs). When it comes to cancer, however, because of the existence of

hormone receptors on most tissues in the body, hormones can influence control over disease processes—but that is different than causing the cancer to start in the first place. In other words, hormones can influence growth of existing cancer but they do not initiate and bring about cancer.

If estrogen were cancer causing and the main driver of breast cancer, we would expect breast cancer rates to decline during menopause, when hormones decline, but the opposite actually occurs. In fact, as women age and lose estradiol, they are more at risk of developing breast cancer. Likewise, if estrogen were cancer causing, we would expect pregnant women to have high rates of cancer because estradiol is at a lifetime high during pregnancy, but, again, the opposite is true. It turns out that pregnancy, with its massive hormone exposure, protects against breast cancer in the long run. In fact, the younger a woman is with her first pregnancy, the more lifelong protection she has while never having a baby actually increases a woman's risk of developing breast cancer by 30 percent.

Sadly, despite decades of research and billions of dollars invested in studying it, the reality is that the exact mechanisms underlying how cancer starts are still not known, but evidence suggests it is changes to our cells' DNA as well as disruptions in their life cycle that cause cancer. To this end, inflammation is strongly associated with the development of cancer and it is widely accepted that estradiol loss, whether surgical or natural, creates an inflammatory state in our bodies from midlife and beyond.

Another influence on cancer comes via the tumor-suppressing protein called p53, which repairs DNA and regulates cell division by keeping cells from growing and dividing too fast or in an uncontrolled

DESPITE THE FEAR-FILLED MESSAGING on estradiol and cancer, there is ample evidence that a paradigm shift from this traditional thinking to a recognition that estradiol, whether made by the body or taken for restoration, actually prevents cancer, and that when the disease does occur, estradiol use leads to earlier detection and significantly reduced mortality.

way. As we describe earlier, the rhythm and peaks of estradiol and progesterone over the twenty-eight days of the female menstrual cycle specifically stimulate the p53 suppressor gene's action. Accordingly, the loss of these hormones and their cyclic rhythms results in a loss of stable action by p53 and an increase in cancer risk. In fact, it is believed that estradiol actually maintains an anti-tumor environment by inhibiting inflammation and helping regulate cell life cycles. In addition to inflammation and deranged life cycles, cancer risk is also increased by the existence of comorbidities such as insulin resistance, metabolic syndrome, poor liver detoxification, and impaired gut health—all things that women are more susceptible to as hormones decline.

Evidence for estradiol's protective effects against cancer can be seen in the statistics. Breast cancers that develop in women using estradiol replacement are smaller, less clinically advanced, have a lower rate of lymph node positivity, are better differentiated, and are of a more favorable type than cancers that develop in women who do not use estradiol replacement. In terms of cancers other than those

of the breast, replacing estradiol actually decreases the risk of recurrence and death from the cancer. Specifically, women colorectal cancer survivors who use estradiol have a lower risk of death from any cause than survivors who do not use estradiol. Similarly, women who are survivors of skin cancer and use estradiol have a longer survival rate than non-estradiol survivors.

We hope all this information enables you to see the critical importance—far beyond fertility—of estradiol and progesterone for women over their entire life span.

The fact is, the menopausal transition is a progressive change from a balanced, healthy state to a state of continuous degeneration that is, in large part, due to the loss of estradiol and progesterone. Although this reality is universal for all women, what is often quite different from woman to woman is whether the transition brings with it physical symptoms, typically hot flashes, night sweats, foggy brain, mood changes, vaginal dryness, low libido, low energy, weight gain, poor sleep, and more. When present, these symptoms can serve as warning signs of the onset of rapid aging and the degenerative processes triggered by hormone loss.

What is critical to know, however, is that not all women have symptoms of hormone decline, or what they do experience they do not connect to their hormones and find them tolerable or temporary. The problem is, even if the symptoms disappear or are not present at all, the continuous degenerative processes continue.

Although many of these "normal" functional declines and the resulting progression of disease have become expected as a process of aging, the studies are clear that it is not simply "just aging" at play and, thus, most of these declines can be significantly prevented or mitigated with correctly implemented hormone restoration. Because changes from hormone loss accumulate over time, women's quality of health dramatically changes every decade after age fifty. For this reason, addressing hormone decline is best started when levels fall outside physiologic ranges into suboptimal ranges—for most women this starts in her forties but can be as early as the thirties. Even if those years went by before a woman realized what was at stake, properly replacing hormones can still be effective and beneficial even when we are in our sixties and seventies. In other words, earlier is best but later has benefits, too. In fact, there is no reason to believe (let alone evidence to support) that we ever need to stop replacing our hormones.

As compelling as the case may be for replacing hormones during and after the menopausal transition, however, two realities exist:

- Hormones need a healthy host.
- Not all women are candidates for hormone restoration.

For this reason, and although we believe that hormone loss should eventually be addressed when possible, it is not *nor should it be* the first tool for women to use when creating a plan to combat the functional declines and to thrive in midlife and beyond. In fact, it is essential that women learn and incorporate nutrition and lifestyle choices targeted for this stage of life with the goal of addressing any and all metabolic, gut, or other health issues first.

Truly aging well and maintaining metabolic health do not happen with one magic button. These things take work and must be intentional and consistent. Although we often hear from women that this is the hardest part, especially because there is a lot of noise and mixed messaging around nutrition and lifestyle practices for women in and past the menopausal transition, we believe a simple and successful template exists that will help you control how you age as you grow older. The strategy to optimize your metabolic health is what we will share next!

PART TWO

HEALTHY AGING THROUGH MIDLIFE AND MENOPAUSE

Optimal Metabolic Health via Nutrition, Gut, Lifestyle, Adrenals, and Thyroid Optimization

CHAPTER FIVE

THE IMPORTANCE OF METABOLIC HEALTH

WE WANT TO START THIS NEXT SECTION by helping you frame what you are about to read as assembling a toolbox for midlife. Inside that toolbox are the foundations of nutrition, movement, sleep, stress reduction, and other areas that need attention, before or concurrent with starting any medical approaches to hormones. Midlife is a time to put your metabolic house in order. You would never invite company over with your house a mess and ill-equipped for guests—hormone therapy and other medical interventions should be seen as guests visiting your home, which you would prep accordingly. In other words, please do not skip ahead to hormone therapy because your body as host needs to have itself in order, ideally first!

When we talk about "metabolic health," we refer to how efficiently the process of metabolism works. In standard terms, metabolism is the process through which cells in our bodies break down the foods we eat and convert them into energy. This definition of metabolism is too simplified, however, because, in reality, metabolism goes beyond simply turning food into energy. Rather, metabolism is the sum and homeostasis of all chemical reactions in your body that keep you alive. This includes not just producing and utilizing energy but also controlling growth and cellular reproduction, building new tissues, breaking down and repairing old tissues, and eliminating waste. When metabolic health is on point, we are free of metabolic diseases, such as diabetes, obesity, and heart disease. When metabolism is dysregulated, metabolic health suffers and disease risk increases.

WHAT IS METABOLIC HEALTH?

Conventional medicine likes to give benchmarks to evaluate metabolic health. Specifically, they have identified the following five characteristics essential for metabolic health:

1 **Waist circumference** of less than or equal to 35 inches (89 cm) for women and less than or equal to 40 inches (102 cm) for men

2 **Fasting blood glucose** of less than or equal to 100 mg/dL

3 **Systolic blood pressure** of lower than 120 mmHg and diastolic blood pressure lower than 80 mmHg

4 **Triglycerides** less than 150 mg/dL

5 **HDL (good) cholesterol** of 50mg/dL in women and above 40mg/dL in men

If someone falls outside of three of these five criteria listed, the diagnosis is "metabolic syndrome," or MetS. Having MetS means having a significantly elevated risk of developing chronic cardiometabolic issues, such as type 2 diabetes, heart disease, and stroke, along with an increased risk for having a reduction in both quality and length of life.

Although clinical guidelines for metabolic health are convenient for doctors, it is not an entirely accurate approach to identify metabolic disease risk. Metabolic health is not a binary "if this, then that" state; instead, metabolic health exists on a spectrum where simply not having a disease diagnosis does not mean someone is healthy. For example, someone might not be clinically obese, but if they have visceral fat or fat stored deep in their belly around their organs, they are not metabolically healthy. Likewise, someone might not have type 2 diabetes, but if they have large or long-lasting swings in blood sugar levels after meals, they are not metabolically healthy.

The other problem with clinical guidelines is that many people "feel fine" and never receive any perceptible warning signs that their health is poor, especially because the symptoms of metabolic dysfunction can go unnoticed or do not show up until a condition is severe. No one can "feel" high triglycerides or low HDL and may not know it is a problem until they develop pancreatitis or have a heart attack. These conditions arise primarily due to poor nutrition, insulin resistance, a sedentary lifestyle, low-quality and inconsistent sleep, unmanaged stress, chronic inflammation, and toxin exposure.

Although some aspects of metabolic health, such as mitochondrial function, are somewhat fixed by age, sex, and genetics, the biggest drivers of metabolic health are actually levers within your control. We may not be able to be twenty again, but we can modify our diet, gut microbiome, weight, sleep, and exercise, and we can address our stress levels and mental health status. For this reason, it is important to remember that whether a disease has been diagnosed and whether you feel or look healthy are somewhat irrelevant. Every day you have a chance to improve your metabolic health and overall health: All it takes is some guidance tailored to midlife.

METABOLIC HEALTH IN MIDLIFE MATTERS: HORMONES NEED A HEALTHY HOST

Metabolic health is uniquely vulnerable to disruption whenever inflammation is present in the body, even low-grade inflammation without any symptoms; it is for this reason that midlife women need to pay attention. As discussed previously, the loss of sex hormones through the menopausal transition and beyond promotes metabolic dysfunction by predisposing women to obesity and abdominal fat, insulin resistance, cardiovascular and lipid changes, chronic inflammation, disrupted sleep, and increased oxidative stress. Because of this, many women think that simply replacing those declining and lost hormones is all that is needed to restore their health. This is not entirely true.

To be sure, women's long-term overall health does rely on the rhythmic cycling of physiologic levels of hormones; however, hormones do not act in a vacuum. By this, we mean that not only do hormones help support a body's health, but they also perform best—in and in fact, require—a healthy body to do so. Studies show that replacing low hormones without first, or at least concurrently, addressing poor metabolic health can increase women's cancer risk, double heart disease risk, and worsen unhealthy inflammation. Additionally, replacing hormones cannot, on its own, restore diminished health to eliminate the immense cardiometabolic burden caused by low hormones in midlife.

While the hormonal changes and health risks of this phase of life can feel a bit overwhelming and deflating, the truth is that all these things are modifiable, and we hold much of the power simply with our daily habits. We tell women that metabolic health

WITH RESPECT TO THE CASCADE of metabolic changes triggered by low hormones, here is a quick recap from previous chapters:

- **Declining estrogen** changes the way our body processes glucose.

- **Impaired glucose** handling leads to insulin resistance.

- **Insulin resistance** leads to increased fat storage, which then also shifts from the hips and thighs to the abdomen, a.k.a. "visceral fat," and visceral fat increases health risks of CVD, type 2 diabetes, and metabolic syndrome.

- **Similarly, declining estrogen** affects the signaling of our "hunger hormones" leptin and ghrelin, and dysfunctional hunger hormones lead to overeating, which leads to more fat and inflammation.

- **Declining testosterone and estrogen** lead to loss of muscle mass, which results in the body swapping fat for muscle, thereby slowing the rate at which we use calories.

- **Slower metabolism** leads to overeating, which leads to inflammation, further impairing bone, heart, and brain health.

- **Declining hormones** disrupt sleep, and poor sleep leads to inflammation, weight gain, and poor stress handling, which then spikes cortisol, triggering more overeating and more fat.

should be viewed as a multipiece puzzle, the completion of which requires us to commit to making daily consistent and intentional actions to ensure all pieces fit together properly. When one piece is missing or in the wrong place, our bodies are put under stress and a cascade of negative health issues develops.

So, how do we ensure that the puzzle is complete and correct? We focus on the basic foundations of health by constructing a pyramid of priorities that restore and nurture our bodies (and minds!) from the inside out. The best part is that these are not complex interventions; in fact, we refer to them as "low-hanging fruit" and, more important, they are accessible to all women.

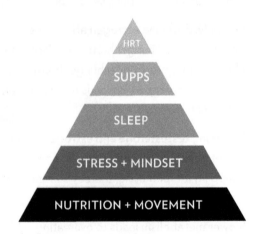

NUTRITION IS THE BIGGEST LEVER TO PROMOTE METABOLIC HEALTH

The single biggest influence we have on our metabolic health is our daily food choices. Proper nutrition can help us achieve a healthy weight, regulate variations in blood sugar and insulin, lower chronic inflammation, improve sleep, and so much more. Although the conventional messaging around nutrition tells us to eat a diet full of healthy unprocessed foods like fruits, vegetables, legumes, seeds and nuts, whole grains, and healthy fats and to limit sweetened drinks, refined grains, and ultra-processed foods, this advice falls short when it comes to women in midlife and beyond.

Declining sex hormones in midlife alter how our bodies handle certain foods compared to in our teens, twenties, and thirties. Alongside our hormone decline is a decline in muscle, in both quantity and quality. While muscle is often thought of as a biomechanical asset in that it helps us with movement, it is also an important bio*chemical* asset in that it supports bone remodeling, helps control inflammatory response, and even modulates the immune system, among other things. For this reason, the combination of low sex hormones and declining muscle means that midlife women need to adjust their nutrition choices to address these two realities. Although the solution is quite simple—eating enough calories and enough of key foods—knowing how and why to eat this way are things many women struggle with.

WHY WE'VE LOST OUR NUTRITION INTUITION

Feeding our bodies to look and perform the way we desire *should* be common sense, or, at the very least, not difficult—but, unfortunately, decades of sparse education, horrible government advice, and constantly shifting messaging on this topic have most of us questioning whether we even possess intuition around nutrition anymore. One of the biggest mind benders for women as they enter the menopausal transition is how seemingly, out of the blue, the nutrition and lifestyle choices that have (ostensibly) served them fine up to this point suddenly no longer work. Many women "see" the changes, with a thicker belly and extra pounds on the scale, whereas some just feel softer, weaker, or less energetic.

No matter when it happens, most women respond to this change by leaning into a "less is more" mindset with respect to food by eating fewer calories and often fewer dietary fats. One of the most popular methods used by women eating less to move the scale is some form of fasting, something we will have a few things to say about later. No matter how it is done, this duo of low-calorie plus low-fat nutrition frequently translates into fewer dense proteins, especially red meat, which often results in muscle loss, anemia (low iron), and/or additional hormone issues—hormones are created from cholesterol and require dietary fat.

On top of eating less, women tend to adopt an almost punitive "more is more" approach with respect to exercise, investing ridiculous amounts of time in cardio-based exercise (High-Intensity Interval Training [HIIT], circuits, endurance work, etc.) with the (very flawed) belief that we can "burn" calories to lose fat or tone up. The combination of less food and more exercise creates a perfect storm that leaves us feeling drained and needing to subsist on "fast energy" caffeine and/or "health-haloed" packaged foods, often high in carbohydrates.

Wound up and stretched at the same time, some women become blind to the stress hormone cortisol coursing through their veins or, worse, routinely reach for an evening glass of wine to "de-stress," only to feel like crud the next day. Wash, rinse, repeat: It is

THE SCALE IS NOT AN ACCEPTABLE MEASURING STICK

ONE IMPORTANT MYTH we would like to put front and center is that the scale should **never** be the sole determinant of a woman's state of health. In our work, we have seen plenty of "thin" women who are prediabetic with high inflammation markers, and we have seen plenty of women 10 to 20 pounds (4.5 to 9 kg) overweight who have beautiful lipids, blood sugar, and inflammation status. Because problems such as insulin resistance and other metabolic disorders develop slowly and move silently, their symptoms may not be apparent until well after negative health changes are entrenched. In addition, there are plenty of health issues triggered or exacerbated by poor nutrition that don't impact the scale, such as poor mood, disrupted sleep, GI issues like bloating and slow bowels, allergies/asthma, liver detox issues, and more. For this reason, thin should not be the goal; *healthy* should be the goal.

a vicious cycle . . . and it seriously impairs women's health by creating an environment of "catabolism," or "breakdown," of our tissues, primarily muscle. Because of the habits typically adopted due to scale chasing, midlife women tend to fit into one of three groups: 1) malnourished from either over- or undereating; 2) "fit" but unhealthy; or 3) healthy but unfit.

Regardless of how a woman loses her intuition on nutrition, low muscle mass and low strength universally dominate as the primary problems driving metabolic issues in midlife. Although this may seem like a daunting problem to overcome, it actually provides the road map needed for how to get our wits and waistline intact once again! By shifting our nutrition and lifestyle choices to those that optimize metabolic health and muscle preservation, we can drastically mitigate the effects of low hormones and set ourselves up to maximally thrive should we choose hormone restoration. Shifting our choices to a nutritional template with macronutrients that are lower in carbohydrates and higher in protein, and not being fearful of fat, gives women the best chance of optimizing health as they enter and travel through the menopausal transition.

MACRONUTRIENTS: THE BASICS

Macronutrients are the three essential nutrients women's bodies need in large quantities on a daily basis to provide energy, prevent disease, and allow their bodies to function with good health. Carbohydrates (or carbs), protein, and fat are the macronutrients in the human diet and are often referred to as "macros." The vast majority of foods contain some of each of the three macronutrients but most often are classified as just one type of macronutrient based on what they contain the most of, for example:

- Beef is a protein
- Avocado is a fat
- Rice is a carb

Each macro has a different "energy," or caloric density, with carbs and protein counting as 4 calories per gram and fat as 9 calories per gram. Although calories matter, different foods affect metabolism differently, with some macros requiring more work to digest, absorb, or metabolize than others. The measure used to quantify this work is called the "thermic effect of food" and the higher the thermic effect, the more energy a food requires to be metabolized. Think of fats, protein, and carbs like wood in a fire. Carbs are like the kindling that burns quickly but needs to be fed more frequently to keep burning. Fats and proteins are the big, thick logs that keep the fire going, burning steadily for hours without needing to be attended to constantly.

Because of these differences, various foods can affect your hormones, hunger, feelings of fullness, and metabolism differently, referred to collectively as satiety, regardless of the number of calories they contain.

SATIETY AND HUNGER ARE THE GOAL

Satiety is driven by hormonal balance, specifically between the hormones leptin and ghrelin, which control appetite and hunger by sending certain signals to our brain. This is called the "neuroregulation of appetite." Think of satiety not as "I feel full" or "this tastes good" but rather as a physical state in which there is no longer a desire to eat. Whether you regularly achieve satiety is easily judged by how long you can go effortlessly without eating between meals (and not relying on caffeine, consuming high volumes of water/fluids, or requiring other energy support). If it is only two to three hours, your current nutrition is not achieving satiety. Ideally, when nutrition is on point, you can last four to six hours between meals.

Although we all start life with a natural regulation of satiety, many of us have broken this system by chronically pursuing certain habits. Specifically, chronic dieting and calorie restriction, eating low-fat foods, consuming low-nutrient, hyperpalatable foods (most often refined grains and carbohydrates), and overeating are the biggest derailers of our leptin and ghrelin balance. Once these hormones are disrupted, their signals become compromised, and the body stops recognizing when we are truly satisfied versus truly hungry.

When this happens, satiety ends up being signaled by a stomach-stretch receptor, which explains why fibrous (bloating) foods (grains and veggies) and liquids (smoothies, copious coffee, or other fluids) leave us "feeling" full (a.k.a. stretched) but only temporarily, because we are hungry and seeking food again within a couple of hours or relying on caffeine and other fake energy sources.

In addition to satiety issues, there are three other types of "hunger" that can drive food-seeking behavior.

1 **Nutrient hunger** happens when nutrition is low in raw materials, usually protein and minerals, and the body attempts to signal this to you.

2 **Energy hunger** happens when nutrition is dependent on fast-burning fuels (carbohydrates) and lacks optimal amounts of slow-burning fuels (protein and fat).

3 **Hedonic hunger** happens when you are not actually hungry but seek food as a form of reward or pleasure (this most often results with a combined carbohydrate and fat food, such as cookies and other treats).

Sometimes we may be up against a combination of more than one type of hunger, and it can be difficult in the moment to identify how to get out of it other than reaching for the nearest convenience food. Thankfully, there is a way to rehab your satiety signals, and all it takes is learning about different fuels and how to craft a nutritional template tailored to midlife. The next chapter provides guidance so you can take satiety *and* your metabolic health into your own hands.

CHAPTER SIX

CURATING NUTRITION FOR MIDLIFE

BECAUSE OF THE METABOLIC CHANGES that come with age, coupled with declining and, ultimately, deficient hormones, nutrition in midlife needs to be different. No longer can we eat the same type and quantity of foods that we ate in our premenopausal years, and this reality hits most women quite hard, leaving them very confused, as if they have lost their basic intuition on what and how to eat.

If you feel you have lost your intuition with nutrition or you are tired of all the mixed messages and noise out there, don't despair! Although all of this information may seem overwhelming (and infuriating), the good news is, recognizing different types of hunger, seeking satiety, and accepting the way that declining hormones change metabolism all go a long way toward helping to reawaken our nutrition intuition. Ultimately, our food choices should be such that they balance blood sugar, optimize for muscle, control inflammation, and mitigate weight gain, which, together, will have the effect of achieving satiety, avoiding hunger, and optimizing your metabolic and overall health. By now, you are likely asking, "*How* do I achieve that?" An incredibly simplified answer is this: Follow a low-carbohydrate, high-(animal) protein, moderate-fat template—but rather than just taking our word for it, let's dig into the specifics.

CARBS: WHY THEY MATTER AND NEED CARE

Carbohydrates, most likely, feel picked on lately as the nutrition world has been experiencing a powerful movement toward cutting carbs from one's diet. Although we will be the first to admit there has been some overcorrection in this regard, for midlife women there is a justification to take a look at your carb intake and do some curating. When women lose estrogen and hormonal rhythms, they lose some of their fine-tuned ability to process carbohydrates the same way they did in their younger years, including even from healthy sources such as unprocessed or minimally processed whole grains, vegetables, fruits, and beans. In addition, carbs are a quick fuel, meaning they rarely drive satiety and require us to continually eat to meet our body's needs. Anyone who has attempted to replace a balanced meal with simply a huge bowl of veggies can attest to this!

Presently, the average Western diet includes 350 to 400 grams of carbs per day. The problem is that physiologically our bodies process only about 40 grams of carbs in any given meal, and carbs eaten in excess of 40 grams in one sitting are sent to the liver and packaged as triglycerides. High triglycerides drive hardening and/or thickening of the arteries, which increases the risk of stroke, heart attack, and heart disease. Additionally, high triglycerides can lead to acute inflammation of the pancreas (pancreatitis) and contribute to the development of metabolic syndrome, or MetS. Given that low sex hormones already predispose midlife women to these conditions, it is important not to throw fuel on the fire by consuming excessive carbohydrates.

Finding Your Carb Threshold

So, how many carbs should you have each day? Technically, given current Western dietary habits that average around 300 grams per day, a "low-carb" template would be anything less than 150 grams per day. Although this may be a good place to start, for some women, the actual amount needs to be tailored to them as an individual and based on their "metabolic flexibility," body composition, and activity level.

Metabolic flexibility refers to whether your body is able to easily switch between fuel sources from different macronutrients such as carbs and fats, and effortlessly go for stretches of four to six hours between meals. Many midlife women are primarily "carb burners," meaning they go from one quick fuel to the next and need to eat throughout the day, snack often, get irritable from hunger, have energy crashes and/or brain fog, and more. Not only is this a miserable way to live as you are subconsciously always focused on your next source of food, but it also increases inflammation and blood sugar dysregulation, thereby impairing metabolic health. The only way to restore or improve metabolic flexibility is to reduce carbs in the diet and "teach" your body to rely on fuel from protein and fat.

Carbohydrate tolerance is also connected to body composition in that muscle tissue acts as an important reservoir, or "sink," for carbohydrates. If you are "undermuscled," meaning that regardless of your scale weight, your lean muscle mass is low, your threshold for carbohydrates will also be low. Likewise, if you have weight to lose in excess of about 15 pounds (7 kg), then your carb intake needs to be low to honor the reality of "oxidative priority," or the body's decision tree for which fuel to burn first (more on that on page 172).

NET CARBS
OR TOTAL CARBS?

————————

SOME INTERNET ADVICE TELLS WOMEN to focus on "net carbs," which means only counting grams of carbs after subtracting any fiber and/or sugar alcohol grams from total carbs. Although about 25 grams of fiber daily can be helpful for gut health, fiber and sugar alcohols generally should not be considered when determining your carb threshold because they are not without calories. For this reason, *focus on total carbs*, not net.

Finally, your daily activity level can help guide your carb threshold. If you are mostly sedentary, your carbohydrate needs are likely quite low. Remember, carbs act as a quick, on-demand fuel, but if you are not moving throughout the day (even if you hit the gym in the morning for an hour, there are still another fifteen waking hours in the day!), you really do not need many carbs. On the flip side, if you are on your feet all day and engage in some intense exercise on top of that, your carb threshold is most likely higher than the typical midlife woman.

Some Simple Guidelines for Carb Targets

An easy way to look at daily carb intake is to assess your current health and activity and then adjust from there. If you:

- Are dealing with blood sugar issues, such as insulin resistance, *and/or* excess fat (more than 20 pounds [9 kg]), then a good threshold is 20 grams per day

- Are insulin sensitive and not entirely metabolically flexible, as in you have difficulty going longer than three hours without food, *and* have 10 to 20 pounds (4.5 to 9 kg) to lose, then a good threshold is less than 50 grams per day

- Have about 10 pounds (4.5 kg) or so to lose, but you are fully metabolically flexible and strongly insulin sensitive, then a good threshold is 75 grams per day

- Do strength training regularly (minimum of three times per week) with 10 pounds (4.5 kg) or fewer to lose, then a good threshold is 75 to 100 grams per day

- Are very disciplined in the gym (strength training more than three times per week), *and* highly active all day long with fewer than 10 pounds (4.5 kg) to lose, then a good threshold is 120 grams per day

Tips for Low-Carb Foods

Finding healthy carbs does not have to be hard. Because of the nutrient value they offer, fruits and veggies are great places to invest when it comes to carbs. That said, know which foods are low in carbs to make the best decisions for you.

- **Fruits:** Berries are best (blackberries, blueberries, raspberries, strawberries), plus cantaloupe, peaches, tart citrus, watermelon

- **Vegetables:** Asparagus, broccoli, cabbage, cauliflower, cucumber, green beans, leafy greens, mushrooms, olives, tomatoes, zucchini

LOW-CARB PITFALLS TO AVOID

Common problems reported with eating "low carb" are that it causes low energy, hair loss, headaches, poor mood, and more. This is often due to being unaware of three common pitfalls that can trigger these issues; however, bolstered with the right information you can avoid them and thrive with low-carb nutrition.

- **Pitfall #1:** When our diet has a low amount of carbohydrates, our blood sugar stays low and so insulin levels are kept low. When insulin is kept low, the kidneys excrete sodium at a faster rate than usual, disrupting the mineral balance in our cells, leading to muscle cramps, fatigue, headaches, and other issues. For this reason, supporting electrolytes is key with low-carb nutrition. Not all electrolytes are created equal, so look for a robust blend of sodium, potassium, and magnesium without added sugars or other unnecessary ingredients.

- **Pitfall #2:** Women often combine low-carb nutrition with low-fat nutrition, which will tank your energy and result in poor-quality food choices— those without enough nutrient density. We're talking steamed veggies and big undressed salads or, worse, convenience foods such as bars marketed as low carb, both of which leave your body undernourished and lead to negative health outcomes.

- **Pitfall #3:** When trying to avoid carbs, many women end up, inadvertently, under-consuming calories because they forget to replace the carbs with another fuel in their diet. When we provide the body with too few calories to meet our metabolic needs, our health becomes impaired. Simply by being mindful to replace those skipped carbs with another fuel—primarily protein—we are sure to get enough calories and support our body's nutritional needs.

PROTEIN: YOUR MISSING PIECE

If we were to give just one bit of advice for what to focus on with nutrition in midlife, it would be to prioritize protein. Due to the changing hormonal landscape in the menopausal transition, midlife women need more, and optimal, protein than at any other time in life due to the loss of muscle as they age.

Protein's Starring Role

Among all the roles protein plays in our body and health, its starring role is in regulating satiety, preserving muscle, and supporting weight loss. Protein triggers hormones that promote feelings of fullness and satisfaction, thereby reducing appetite and preventing overeating. In fact, it has been found that people were likely to eat around 441 fewer calories per day and feel more satisfied when protein made up more than 30 percent of their diet.

Additionally, protein causes the largest rise in the thermic effect of food, meaning the body burns more calories digesting protein compared to fat or carbs. Specifically, protein increases your metabolic rate by 15 to 30 percent, compared to 5 to 10 percent for carbs and 0 to 3 percent for fats. Because of this, eating more protein reduces the drop in metabolism often associated with losing fat because it reduces muscle loss and muscle is needed to maintain metabolic energy.

Finally, prioritizing protein keeps us strong as we age. In studies of older women, consuming more than 1.1 grams of protein per pound (455 g) of body weight every day was linked to a decreased risk of frailty, a condition marked by weakness, loss of strength, and other changes that often occur during the aging process.

Not All Protein Is Created Equal

Dietary proteins are made up of chemical building blocks called amino acids, and these molecules are used to build and repair muscles and bones and to make the hormones and enzymes responsible for triggering many of our biological processes. Protein can also be used as an energy source. To influence metabolism and protect muscle, dietary protein must satisfy three requirements:

1 Quantity
2 Quality
3 Distribution

PROTEIN QUANTITY

As we age, our muscles experience something called "anabolic resistance," which means they become less responsive to the stimulus from dietary protein. In addition to aging, anabolic resistance is also increased by the rapid loss of sex hormones and the ensuing chronic low-grade inflammation during the menopausal transition. Because of this, women start losing muscle in their thirties and experience a rapid increase of muscle loss in the decades that follow. What this means is that by midlife, women must consume more protein to support their muscle health than they had to eat in their youth.

PROTEIN QUALITY

It is not merely enough to increase the amount of protein in our diet; rather, it is important to pay attention to the type, or quality, of protein as well. The *quality* of dietary protein is determined by three factors:

1 **Completeness of its amino acid profile:** Dietary proteins contain twenty common amino acids, nine of which are "essential" and must be present and consumed for optimal health.

2 **Whether its amino acids provide cellular stimulus:** Certain amino acids used for cell-specific production of metabolites with enormous physiological importance must be present.

3 **Digestibility and nutrient bioavailability:** It is essential that the nutrients in the protein are broken down and absorbed easily by the body.

Two types of protein exist: plant protein and animal protein. When evaluated for quality, *only animal protein* adequately meets all three factors.

Plant proteins lack key essential amino acids, contain nutrients requiring complex conversion in the gut and certain "antinutrients" that block the protein's digestion and absorption, and provide low to no amounts of the amino acids needed for cellular stimulus to muscle preservation. For example, grains and legumes are deficient in the essential amino acid lysine, whereas fruits and vegetables often lack methionine. When the body lacks an amino acid in the diet, it will break down muscle to release that missing amino acid. Similarly, the digestibility and bioavailability of plant proteins are lower due to the presence of antinutritional factors, such as phytates and protease inhibitors, which can inhibit protein absorption.

Animal protein, however, provides a complete and optimal amino acid profile and is particularly stimulating for muscle remodeling; contains preformed, bioavailable nutrients that need no conversion and are easily digested and absorbed; and has aminos that protect against inflammation and oxidative stress. In addition, animal protein is the only source

THE PLANT-BASED PROBLEM

NOT MUCH IN THE NUTRITION WORLD is as polarizing as the conversation around animal versus plant-based proteins. Ardent followers of plant-based nutrition insist it is possible to "prepare" plant proteins (such as soaking and sprouting them) to make them more digestible and to combine plant proteins to reach amino acid goals. Unfortunately, when it comes to targeting optimal metabolic health by prioritizing protein for muscle preservation, not only do plants—however prepared and combined—still fall short, but they also come packaged with a significant amount of carbohydrates, which create their own problems, and will still require additional supplementation of missing vitamins and minerals. To demonstrate this, let's compare black beans to beef.

Black Beans	Beef
2 cups (340 g) cooked black beans	6 ounces (170 g) beef steak
Calories = 437 kcal	Calories = 150 kcal
Protein = 30 grams	Protein = 42 grams
Carbs = 88 grams	Carbs = 0 grams
Optimal Amino Acids = No	Optimal Amino Acids = Yes
Bioavailable Iron = No	Bioavailable Iron = Yes
Vitamin B_{12} Present = No	Vitamin B_{12} Present = Yes
Antinutrients = Yes	Antinutrients = No

of key vitamins and minerals that plant proteins do not provide, specifically vitamins B_{12}, D_3, E, and K_2, as well as minerals like zinc and heme iron.

PROTEIN DISTRIBUTION

When it comes to eating protein, women typically tend to skew their intake with low amounts at breakfast, slightly more at lunch, and the largest amount at dinner. This pattern is problematic because an uneven distribution increases anabolic resistance and impairs appetite control, satiety, gut health, and weight management. In addition, our muscles are most primed to benefit from protein intake first thing in the morning, when we are coming off our overnight fast. For this reason, to best benefit from dietary protein, midlife women need to spread their protein intake evenly among meals and should add supplemental protein after strength training to "feed" muscles.

Setting a Protein Target

Just as with carbohydrates, you may be wondering what your protein target should be and, thankfully, it is relatively easy to calculate. Considering low hormones and anabolic resistance, to achieve the minimum amount of amino acids required to preserve muscle, eat *at least* 35 grams of protein at each of three meals per day. Ideally, consume protein each day that equates to 1 gram per pound (or 2.2 grams per kilogram) of ideal body weight. So, if you are targeting a scale weight of 140 pounds (63.5 kg), you want to aim for 140 grams of protein each day, ideally primarily from animal sources and evenly distributed among breakfast, lunch, and dinner. Not only will you have better satiety and balanced

energy, but you will also improve your bones, muscle, inflammation, and overall health!

Tips to Get Optimal Protein

If shifting your nutrition to achieve these protein targets seems overwhelming, we have some helpful suggestions:

- **Mix and layer proteins:** Get more "bang for your buck" by combining different proteins, such as a couple of scallops with your steak or shrimp with your burger.

- **Avoid palate fatigue:** Embrace clean, premade seasoning blends to add variety, and experiment with different types and cuts of meat.

- **For simplicity, choose ground meats:** Ground meats are quick to cook and generally cost less than steaks or other "fancier" cuts.

- **Batch cook:** Because protein sources tend to be the most time-intensive in the kitchen, pick one day each week to batch cook some of your favorite high-protein recipes for easy meals on busy days. Some of our favorites include sloppy Joes, chicken tenders, tuna or salmon salad, roasted salmon, shrimp, and scallops.

- **Buy in bulk:** Once you get the hang of planning and shopping for meals, you'll know how much chicken, fish, eggs, or beef you'll need. Shopping in bulk means saving money per ounce (28 g) of food.

- **Don't eat breakfast for breakfast:** Morning tends to be the hardest time for women to eat ample protein, so shift your idea of what breakfast needs to look like. An easy solution is to make extra food at dinner to reheat in the morning.

- **Reexamine your eating patterns:** Notice the meals and snacks in which you tend to concentrate your protein intake, and the ones in which you don't. How can you shift to expand?

- **Close gaps with high-quality protein powder:** Use a high-quality protein powder or meal replacement once a day if convenience dictates, but do not make this a stand-in for real food.

FAT: YOUR GOLDILOCKS TOOL FOR SATIETY

Like protein, fats are an incredible source of long-burning, steady energy and help balance blood sugar. Beyond that, dietary fats are also essential for whole body health due to their many other roles, such as making up and enabling the absorption of the fat-soluble vitamins A, D, E, and K; making up every cell membrane in the entire body; forming and supporting the function of every hormone; producing healthy cholesterol and bile for proper liver function; protecting and lining organs and joints; and managing the inflammation process. (We also know that healthy fats make foods taste great!)

Although fats are essential for satiety and good health, we want to be completely transparent here and state that we are not fans of keto, or any diets that prioritize high fat intake (and/or constantly being in ketosis), for midlife women. Although these diets have phenomenal therapeutic utility, such as for treating severe depression and other mental health disorders or for managing conditions like seizure disorders and certain cancers, they are not a nutritional template that serves this phase of a woman's life.

Eating primarily fat can drive up stress hormones and lead to excessive caloric intake and weight gain. Conversely, the opposite can also happen. Because fat is so satiating, some women will actually undereat other foods, especially protein, and inadvertently shift their body composition to low muscle volume as the scale moves lower. Given that muscle provides critical biomechanical and biochemical benefits, this is concerning. Finally, many "keto-focused" diets pay zero mind to food quality, so women eat packaged foods labeled "keto" that are full of low-quality ingredients and provide no nutritional value.

Fine-Tuning with Fat

Consider fat as a lever you can tweak up or down as your health, needs, and goals require. For example, if after two weeks of intentionally meeting macros, you have new onset sleep disruption or feel sluggish with exercise, then your fat might be too low. If you feel like you cannot meet your protein goals—the most important—then your fat might be too high. In terms of initial guidance on a macro threshold for fat, usually something around 60 percent of your protein goal is a good starting point. For example, if your protein goal is 140 grams, set your fat goal around 85 grams and add carbs according to the chart on page 78. If you feel that is too few calories, play

FAT SHOULD NOT BE THE FOCUS

AS A REFRESHER, the ultimate goal for the original keto diet was to achieve ketosis. Ketosis occurs when your body starts using fat as its main fuel source due to limited access to glucose, or blood sugar, typically caused by starvation, fasting, or following a very, very low-carb diet.

Clinically, ketosis is a metabolic state in which your blood has a high concentration of ketones, namely beta-hydroxybutyrate. Ketones are a by-product produced when your body uses only fat, instead of glucose, for energy, and can be measured using a ketone monitor and urine or blood. When ketones accumulate in the blood, the body enters ketosis. Ketones are not harmful in small amounts and, for certain medical conditions, being in ketosis persistently is essential—for the average woman, however, it is not. In fact, ketosis itself is a fleeting state and this raises one of our concerns with it. As women become "fat adapted" or metabolically flexible, their ketone levels drop because the body is using them for fuel. This often results in women "chasing" ketones, by focusing solely on consuming dietary fats simply to hit ketone numbers on their monitors.

Although not fans of keto, we are huge fans of dietary fat itself and feel that too many women "fear" fat. Fat is an incredibly important macronutrient for midlife that enables you to fine-tune your energy, performance, mental clarity, mood, and body composition goals; however, it is something you want to leverage *after* hitting your protein goals. Without a doubt, fat is a bit of a "Goldilocks" macro in that, as you've just seen, amounts both too high and too low can create issues.

around with increasing your protein and fat until you find a set point that addresses satiety, energy, sleep, performance, and body composition.

YOU CANNOT MANAGE WHAT YOU DO NOT MEASURE

We have been advising women with respect to nutritional macros for a very long time and it is very common to meet some resistance against having to be intentional with eating for macro targets. We understand. We had our own frustrations with it, too, but to be frank, we have to make change to get change, and when it comes to midlife nutrition, something usually needs tweaking.

Learning to make intentional choices around food does not have to mean measuring, weighing, and tracking every food. Although that may be a helpful method for some, it can feel or become very disordered for others. For this reason, we want you simply to commit to becoming familiar with macro-nutrients by taking five to seven days to log what you regularly eat into an app like Cronometer or MyFitnessPal while simultaneously noting (in the app, a journal, your phone, whatever) how you feel and how your energy, mood, sleep, digestion, and bowels respond. Then, look back at your entries to review things. For example, when you felt an energy slump, how much protein, fat, and carbs had you eaten in the two meals prior? When you felt great and breezed through a day, what macros had you eaten?

Similarly, what were your macros when your belly bloated or your bowels slowed? When you felt some anxiety? When you had poor sleep? And so on.

Your goal is not to micromanage yourself around food but rather to notice trends and be able to dial in what works for you on particular days. Reframe logging food more as a journaling exercise to create a record for yourself that connects food with outcomes. Every woman we have had the pleasure to help has noted how useful this exercise is in learning to visualize what her body is seeking for better health. To get you started, we offer an easy meal template:

AN EASY MEAL TEMPLATE

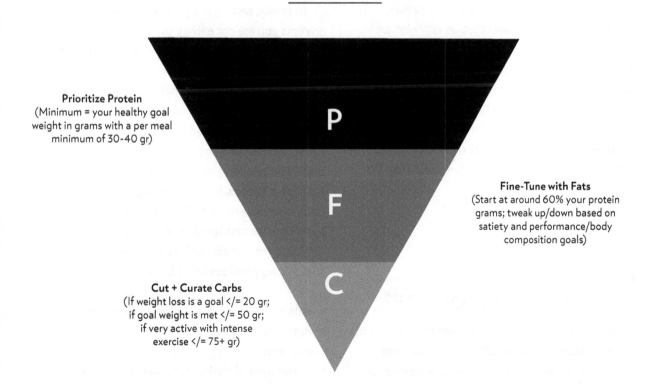

Prioritize Protein
(Minimum = your healthy goal weight in grams with a per meal minimum of 30-40 gr)

P

Fine-Tune with Fats
(Start at around 60% your protein grams; tweak up/down based on satiety and performance/body composition goals)

F

Cut + Curate Carbs
(If weight loss is a goal </= 20 gr; if goal weight is met </= 50 gr; if very active with intense exercise </= 75+ gr)

C

Even after ditching processed foods and eating nutrient-dense whole foods in the proper macronutrient amounts, some women may still have trouble losing fat and managing weight. In these instances, it is important to learn about (and honor) the concept of oxidative priority. This concept is new to many midlife women and, for that reason, we have chosen to explore it more in depth in appendix A (page 172). Please spend some time with it when ready, as it is a crucial piece to the puzzle of weight loss for many women.

WOMEN OFTEN TELL US that their nutrition is fine because they eat "paleo" or "organic" or "clean," etc., which are fine in terms of food quality but can still be problematic overall. Nutrition templates focused only on quality are blind to achieving macronutrient targets, can often be very high carb and low protein, and can even be low fat. Additionally, food manufacturers use these descriptive labels to put a "health halo" on foods that, honestly, are not all that healthy. For this reason, focus on achieving specific macronutrient thresholds using whole, unprocessed, nutrient-dense food sources rather than worrying about whether something fits into a food quality category.

FASTING: FRIEND OR FOE?

For the past few years (and we suspect for the future as well), fasting has been all the rage, but what is it really? Is it the magical fairy for midlife women that it has been made out to be? First, let's distinguish between starvation and fasting, with the difference being a matter of control:

- **Starvation**, outside of an eating disorder, is the involuntary absence of food for a long time, which can lead to suffering or illness and is neither deliberate nor controlled.

- **Fasting** is the voluntary withholding of food for spiritual, health, weight loss, and other reasons. Done correctly, fasting should not cause suffering and is very controlled; food is easily available but you choose not to eat it. Fasting has no standard duration, as it is merely the absence of eating.

In reality, fasting is a part of everyday life because anytime you are not eating, such as overnight to breakfast, you are intermittently fasting. As a tool for weight loss or weight management, fasting allows the body to use its stored energy—that is, burn fat—something very relevant for many midlife women who have chronically followed the all-too-common advice to eat upon waking and then eat every three hours thereafter, resulting in a constant state of being "fed." In these instances, hunger cues are hijacked and the body is never without fuel, so fasting can logically be beneficial because it will break this cycle.

Aside from reducing fuel, many women report that fasting provides other benefits, such as:

- Balanced blood sugar (lower diabetes risk)
- Better balance of hunger hormones (ghrelin and leptin)
- Better mental clarity less brain fog

- Better mood (improves anxiety, depression, stress)
- Gut healing
- Immune system support
- Improved cellular aging (autophagy)
- Improved insulin sensitivity
- Lower risk of heart disease and metabolic syndrome
- Metabolism reset
- Reduced inflammation

Although these sound like great reasons to consider fasting, studies show that it is not that fasting itself is magic but rather that caloric reduction is very powerful for improving metabolic health. By consuming only the fuel we need, we can restore proper hunger signaling, lose weight (sometimes), and balance our health.

The reason we note that fasting only sometimes results in weight loss is because while fasting may help those who struggle with eating too often, it does have some downsides that need to be considered. Many midlife women have the opposite problem from eating too often and actually do not eat enough! At its best, this looks like coffee with collagen for breakfast (coffee is not a food or a meal, so please do not do this), a salad for lunch with a small amount of chicken or other low-fat protein, and an abundance of vegetables and a side portion of

FORMS OF FASTING

Fasting comes in different forms, and the most popular are:

- **5:2 fasting** involves eating 500 to 600 calories for two days out of the week and eating normally the other five days.

- **Alternate-day fasting** is fasting every other day, either by not eating anything or by eating only a few hundred calories.

- **Extended fasting** equals 24 to 72 continuous fasting hours, with liquids only.

- **Eat stop eat** is an intermittent fasting program with one or two 24-hour fasts per week.

- **Intermittent fasting** involves eating two or three meals in a window of 8 to 10 hours during the day, such as between 10 a.m. and 6 p.m, and fasting the remaining 16 to 14 hours; this is also called 16:8 or 14:10.

- **OMAD or warrior diet** means you eat one large meal per day, or only small amounts of vegetables and fruits per day with one huge meal at night.

protein for dinner. At its worst, breakfast is skipped, lunch looks like a snack, and dinner is hit or miss.

Undereating both calories and animal protein creates physiological stress. Not only will this stall any weight loss goals, but it may actually lead to gaining weight as the body adapts to the stress. In addition, eating too little will lead to muscle loss, which not only decreases your strength and fitness but, because muscle is the tissue that utilizes the most calories, also further slows your metabolism.

When you eat too little, your ability to burn off the food you consume declines—and you store the calories as fat. Meanwhile, undereating can also cause your body to start churning out more of the hormones that drive hunger and diminish those involved in satiety, which may lead to binge eating. Undereating can also cause disrupted sleep (from stress and blood sugar issues), make the thyroid struggle (due to a lack of nutrients), and impair hormone production (not enough fat for synthesis). Finally, if you exercise intensely, fasting is not an intervention to consider. Beyond maybe some light cardio, working out without fuel is counterproductive because muscle maintenance is impaired and this can exacerbate body composition and metabolic health problems.

Unless you truly struggle with overeating, we are "Team Three Meals a Day," sometimes with a snack. In reality, no one "needs" to fast and, for that reason, we recommend no more than a twelve- to fourteen-hour fast between the last food of the day and the first meal of the next morning. If you have fasted and feel it "works" for you, that's great, but it is likely due to keeping your calories within a certain limit, and we want to remind you that the same outcome can be had without fasting!

MIDLIFE NUTRITION IN A NUTSHELL

Although this chapter serves up some complex information, midlife nutrition, briefly, is simple: Make satiety your goal to control hunger, lose weight, and improve health.

- Prioritize (animal) protein
- Fine-tune with fat
- Curate and control carbs
- Fast if it fits you

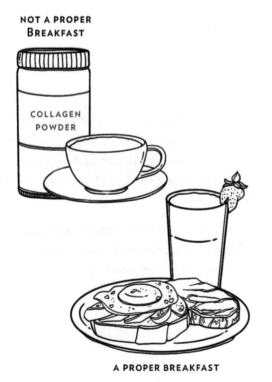

NOT A PROPER BREAKFAST

COLLAGEN POWDER

A PROPER BREAKFAST

By increasing protein and eliminating most carbs from your diet, you eliminate states of high insulin, decrease blood glucose, control inflammation, and use your body's fat to fuel higher energy levels. With a focus on the right macros and nutrients for midlife, you will optimize your hormones, decrease hunger, achieve a healthy weight, and improve your metabolic health.

Incorporating the nuances of midlife nutrition might take a little time and practice, but eventually the stable energy, balanced blood sugar, and improved mood will become easy guideposts that consistently help you correct course when needed.

With nutrition demystified, the next area in which residual issues frequently exist due to loss of hormones is the microbiome. Knowing how to support it in midlife and beyond is just as foundational as nutrition and what we'll explore next.

CHAPTER SEVEN

THE MICROBIOME IN MIDLIFE

Why Daily Poops Are Essential

WHILE NUTRITION IS, WITHOUT A DOUBT, the biggest lever you have to influence your metabolic health in midlife, nutrition is actually more than what we eat. In fact, we must be able to break down and absorb the nutrients in whatever food is consumed. This outcome is entirely dependent on having robust digestion as well as a healthy microbiome. Understanding how digestion works and how to support the microbes in the gut is crucial not just for metabolic but also overall health.

DIGESTION: IT DOESN'T START IN THE MOUTH

The goal of digestion is to reduce food down to molecules so small that the nutrients can be absorbed and used by the cells of the body. Nutrient availability influences everything from mood to weight to our physical experience with hormone replacement therapy. Having good digestion to extract nutrients from the foods and drinks we consume is essential for good health. Although most people think digestion starts in the mouth when we chew our food, it actually starts in the brain where the sight, sound, and smell of food critically triggers everything downstream.

Once food is put into the mouth and chewing begins, oral glands release saliva that contains enzymes that target carbohydrates so they get predigested, leaving less work for the stomach and small intestine. Once food is swallowed, it passes through the esophagus into the stomach where protein digestion should begin. The stomach exposes the food to highly acidic juices designed not just to break down dense protein but also to break down carbs and fats as well as to kill pathogens that might be present. This acid is so strong that to keep it in the stomach, a little flap, or sphincter, at the bottom of the esophagus opens and closes as food comes down based on the acid level detected. Once the stomach's acidity level is optimal, the contents move into the small intestine where various signals are sent to other digestive players.

In the small intestine, more organs join in, with the pancreas releasing bicarbonate to neutralize the bile and enzymes for more nutrient breakdown, and the gallbladder releases bile from the liver to emulsify fats. The breakdown of all nutrients continues until they are ready to be absorbed through the walls of the small intestine and travel via the bloodstream and lymphatic system throughout the body as needed. Whatever remains is sent to the large intestine for one last chance to be recycled before the remaining waste is eliminated as stool. At this point, digestion is complete. Although digestion should be a bodily function on autopilot, a handful of issues can hijack it and impair the process.

Digestion Disruptors

The most common disruptor is exactly where digestion starts: the brain. The entire digestive cascade requires the brain and body to be in a state of rest and relaxation. If we are stressed, rushed, eating on the go, upset, or distracted, the needed stimulatory signals from the brain are not sent and nutrient absorption is minimized. Practicing good mealtime hygiene and mind-set is incredibly effective at optimizing digestion. Some simple tips to ensure a "rest to digest" state are to sit down with your food, take some deep breaths, and pause to give gratitude before starting a meal.

The next digestion hijacker is a lack of chewing. When we eat too fast and, effectively, inhale our food, we impair the release of salivary enzymes and, ultimately, send molecules of food down to the stomach that are too large. One of our favorite tips to avoid this is to practice putting down your utensils between bites of food. Don't pick up your fork or spoon again until your last mouthful has been chewed and swallowed. Practicing deliberate "overchewing" can easily make slower eating a habit and will likely teach you how "fast-paced" your eating has been!

The next most important and yet most maligned contributor to good digestion is stomach acid. Despite advertisements for supplements and medications that claim otherwise, 90 percent of Americans actually do not have enough stomach acid. In his groundbreaking book *Why Stomach Acid Is Good for You*, Jonathan Wright explains how stomach acid is a key essential link in the chain of digestion and that, for too long, we have been unfairly blaming it for digestive problems. Wright explains that a very acidic pH is needed to close the esophageal sphincter and keep the gastric juices from leaving the stomach. When stomach acid is too low, we end up with symptoms such as heartburn, bloating, and burping. This environment actually paves the way for pathogenic infections, leaky gut, poor bile flow, autoimmunity, irritable bowel, and more. Focusing on relaxing the brain, chewing slowly, and avoiding excess fluids at mealtime are all great ways to maximize stomach acid, but if you continue to struggle, then leaning on things like digestive bitters before meals or digestive enzymes during a meal are other options to consider.

An often overlooked obstacle to good digestion is having poor bile flow. Made by the liver and stored in the gallbladder, bile is responsible primarily for emulsifying fats to make them absorbable. To this end, bile also helps with absorption of vitamins A, D, E, and K and aids in waste excretion. The quality and flow of bile can become impaired by a variety of things, from an overworked liver (taxed by alcohol, medications, and toxins) and eating fried foods to low-fat diets, low stomach acid, and chronic stress. Signs of impaired bile include upper right abdominal pain, morning nausea, dry and itchy skin, gallstones, and flat, floating, or greasy stools. Eating healthy fats, and supporting liver health with detoxification supportive teas, castor oil packs over the liver, and ox bile supplements, can work to rehabilitate low-quality or sluggish bile.

Digestion is often described as a "use it or lose it" proposition, meaning that if we let it become diminished, we may struggle long term unless we work to restore it. If you're not sure whether your digestion is on point, an easy trick is to check your poop! Bowel habits are a good indicator of digestive health. Stool color, shape, texture, and buoyancy can indicate problems such as not digesting fats, digestive distress, infection, and, rarely, more serious problems such as cancer. In addition, straining, urgency, or skipping poops are also flags to look out for. Ideally you're pooping once or twice a day with a healthy-looking stool. If you are not sure what that looks like, use the Bristol stool chart with a goal of a regular 3 or 4.

BRISTOL STOOL CHART

Type 1		Separate hard lumps, like nuts (hard to pass)
Type 2		Sausage-shaped but lumpy
Type 3		Like a sausage but with cracks on its surface
Type 4		Like a sausage or snake, smooth and soft
Type 5		Soft blobs with clear-cut edges (passed easily)
Type 6		Fluffy pieces with ragged edges, a mushy stool
Type 7		Watery, no solid pieces—entirely liquid

HOW POOP RELATES TO HORMONES

In 2007, the National Institutes of Health launched the Human Microbiome Project (HMP) in an effort to better understand the vast population of microbiota affecting human health and disease. The HMP figured out that we have ten times as many bacteria, viruses, fungi, and protozoa—collectively known as the microbiome—living on and in us as there are human cells. Essentially, we are more a collection of bacteria than we are cells, and this microbiome performs a critical role in maintaining human health and avoiding disease.

When digestion is impaired, our microbiome shifts away from a balanced, robust, and diverse population of bacteria, resulting in what is known as "dysbiosis." Not only can dysbiosis interfere with the absorption of key nutrients and minerals from our food but it has also been connected to chronic conditions like asthma, cardiovascular disease, chronic kidney disease, diabetes, eczema, inflammatory bowel disease (IBD), irritable bowel syndrome (IBS), liver disease, obesity, rheumatoid arthritis, and even mood and mental health disorders.

As was discussed in chapter 3, estrogen has profound effects on the gut microbiome by maintaining diversity of bacteria and avoiding dysbiosis. The estrobolome within the gut microbiome, likewise, has a strong influence over how our body handles estrogen. This two-way cross talk ensures that a proper amount—not too much, not too little—of estrogen can be detoxed and excreted from the body and that the diversity and volume of our microbiome is health protective. For this reason, whether we are making hormones or taking hormones, it is critical to have daily bowel movements to excrete estrogen and other waste products in a timely manner.

Given that low estradiol can contribute to the same chronic conditions as a poor microbiome, the menopausal transition is a critical time for midlife women to pay attention to the gut. Lack of gastrointestinal symptoms does not mean all is well. Metabolic changes, including increased belly fat, inflammation, high cholesterol, and blood sugar dysregulation, can all be linked to problems with digestion, the microbiome, and the stool.

PROTECTING YOUR MICROBIOME AND OVERALL HEALTH IN MIDLIFE

The loss of estrogen and subsequent changes in the gut microbiota are significant factors driving the whole body health changes that occur in the menopausal transition and beyond. Although a stool test can help identify whether your digestion and microbiome need support, there are some easy habits and interventions that all midlife women should follow.

Include foods that support digestion and microbial diversity. Fermented foods such as yogurt, sauerkraut, kimchi, and kefir can help with the microbiome, and teas such as chamomile, dandelion root, ginger, milk thistle, and peppermint can aid digestion. For proper amounts of β-glucuronidase, the enzyme that keeps estrogen detoxification in check, eating citrus fruits, cruciferous vegetables (like broccoli and arugula), and berries will help.

Avoid foods and drinks that harm your gut. Alcohol, excess caffeine, excess carbonated beverages, fried foods, gluten, sugar alcohols, and sugar-filled and processed foods can inflame the gut lining, disrupt your microbiome, and downregulate digestion. If a food or drink is non-nutritive, meaning it does not provide any helpful nutrients for your health, significantly limit its inclusion in your nutrition choices to protect both your gut and your health.

Consider fiber as Goldilocks. Fiber-rich foods include fruits, vegetables, whole grains, legumes, nuts, and seeds. Fiber is spoken about in hallowed terms, as if it will solve all gut issues. Unfortunately, despite the many claims, there is much more nuance to this topic.

In a large examination of studies on fiber, it has been shown that although dietary fiber can increase the size and volume of bowel movements, it does not improve stool consistency, frequency, or pain, nor does it reduce laxative use or improve constipation treatment outcomes. What this means is that although fiber is important for the microbiome because it provides fuel for our gut microbes, too much fiber can actually back us up. For this reason, be mindful of your fiber intake: Make note of how your bowels respond and adjust accordingly.

Manage hydration. Just like fiber, hydration has a bit of a "not too much, not too little" element to it. Although excess fluids around mealtime can impair the work of gastric juices and reduce good digestion, too little hydration along with diuretics are a problem for bowel movement frequency, which disrupts the microbiome. Because the large intestine pulls minerals and water out of the food we eat, it can make stools hard to pass if we don't provide additional fluid and electrolytes outside of our food. For this reason, being mindful to include minerals with proper hydration is key to a healthy gut.

Keep yourself moving. A sedentary lifestyle and fat- and sugar-rich diets impair the gut and promote obesity; when combined with low estrogen levels, they make midlife women highly susceptible to weight gain and belly fat. This, in turn, promotes unhealthy oxidized cholesterol levels, hypertension, and insulin resistance, which all add up to reduced vitality and poor aging. For this reason, regular daily physical movement is key for regular bowel movements and overall health!

Consider gentler foods when stress is high. Given the brain-bowels connection, managing stress is critical to keeping your gut happy. If your stress is more than what practicing a regular mealtime mind-set and hygiene can overcome, consider some simple food swaps to lighten the load on your strained gut. Switch to ground meats rather than steaks, roasted veggies rather than raw, and berries over whole-flesh fruits, and limit nuts, seeds, and legumes. By giving your digestive system a bit of a reprieve from dense foods, you can support your gut while you address your stress.

Don't overlook digestive and gut supplements. The pancreas naturally produces enzymes to help us break down and absorb nutrients from food, but some people have difficulty making or using those natural enzymes. Whatever is impairing your digestion or gut health, do not overlook some form of supplemental support. One of the safest and most effective options is a basic product providing amylase, protease, and lipase, along with bromelain and papain. If you have special needs, such as problems digesting dairy, gluten, or other similar issues, choose a supplement tailored to support that. Just be mindful that many digestive supplements include additional ingredients that may or may not be right for you. If you are not sure, stick to the basics, or consider stool testing to help tailor digestive support options that are right for you.

Lean on GI support when traveling. Although "traveler's diarrhea" is a well-known phenomenon, "traveler's constipation" is less discussed. To our knowledge, no study has been conducted to evaluate whether traveling is truly associated with constipation, but it is widely reported by many travelers, and we have personally experienced it. The constipation that appears (or worsens) when traveling is usually attributed to changes in diet, hydrating less frequently, following a different meal timetable, and problems finding a bathroom as needed. Also, because the brain and gut are so tightly connected, it has been speculated that jet lag slows bowel movements through this brain-gut axis. Regardless of what you may or may not use when at home, packing digestive enzymes and probiotics can help blunt the effects of travel on your bowels. Additionally, try not to underhydrate simply because you are on the go. While schedule differences may be hard to avoid, being mindful of your food and drink choices while away can go far in keeping your gut and bowels happy, thereby making sure you have a great travel experience.

Be mindful of disruptions from over-the-counter and prescription medications. Constipation caused by medications is, unfortunately, an extremely common and often overlooked condition in midlife. As women age through the menopausal transition, they become more vulnerable to "polypharmacy," or the simultaneous use of multiple medications for one or more conditions. Sadly, this "medication for every symptom" approach ignores the impact it has on the gut. The drugs known to commonly cause constipation include:

- Antibiotics
- Antihistamines
- Antinausea medicines
- Blood pressure medications
- Iron supplements
- Nonsteroidal anti-inflammatory drugs (NSAIDs)
- Opioid pain relievers
- Tricyclic antidepressants
- Urinary incontinence medications

Although nutrition and lifestyle interventions are often able to reduce the reliance on multiple medications, it may not be possible to stop or reduce every drug and thus the lingering side effects on your bowels. In those instances, it is key to incorporate all of the recommendations here for optimizing digestion and protecting your microbiome and overall health to offset these effects.

While nutrition and gut health are the most impactful foundations to focus on in your midlife toolbox, there are other basics that combine to provide equally important support for your whole body health. Key tools include incorporating proper physical movement, practicing stress management, and adopting a mind-set of grace for your changing body and life that happen during midlife and beyond. We will touch on each of these in the chapter ahead.

CHAPTER EIGHT

LIFESTYLE FOUNDATIONS IN MIDLIFE

Adapting the Pillars of Sleep, Stress Management, Movement, Community, and Mind-Set

WHILE NUTRITION AND GUT HEALTH ARE, HANDS DOWN, the biggest levers we have to improve our metabolic health, the daily lifestyle choices we make around sleep, stress management, movement, community, and mind-set are incredibly foundational as well. Of those, quality sleep seems to be the most elusive in midlife and this, unfortunately, almost always leads to problems managing the other lifestyle foundations, resulting in metabolic health decline even with nutrition and gut health on point.

SLEEP, WHERE ART THOU?

We often hear midlife women label themselves a "night owls," with the belief that staying up late and not sleeping well are normal for this stage of life. Common, sure, but normal, no. As humans we have a critical twenty-four-hour internal clock running in the background of our brain that cycles between sleep and activity at regular intervals directed by sunlight. This is called our "circadian rhythm" and it follows a diurnal pattern, meaning we are naturally awake and active during the day, not at night. This rhythm not only controls our sleep/wake cycle but also ensures that important physiological processes are performed at optimal times.

When a body is misaligned with its circadian rhythm, whether episodically or chronically, metabolic health suffers due to the fact that internal organs such as the heart, brain, gut, and more are all tuned to this rhythm. Regardless of lifestyle, people who stay up late have higher levels of body fat, lower levels of muscle mass, dysregulated blood sugar management, disrupted hormone secretions, higher blood pressure, and inverted cortisol secretions compared to those who honor their internal clock. The result for night owls is an overall dramatic increased risk for insulin resistance, hyperglycemia, obesity, diabetes, hypertension, and CVD over time.

Metabolic health is not the only thing impaired by poor sleep. Staying awake too late reduces sleep quality, too, which sets the stage for unhealthy habits during the day, such as being sedentary, drinking alcohol, and indulging in late-night snacks. For these reasons, depression rates tend to be higher for night owls than others.

For women in the menopausal transition and beyond, sleep disturbances usually worsen or appear

CIRCADIAN RHYTHM DISRUPTORS AND GOOD SLEEP HYGIENE

THE MOST COMMON DISRUPTORS to circadian rhythm are:

- Blood sugar problems.
- Ignoring our body's cues directing hunger, sleep, and more.
- Poor liver health.
- Shift work or working at night.
- Stimulation by artificial light close to bedtime.
- Stress (emotional or physiological).
- Time zone travel.

Although some of these disruptors may not be within your control, consistently practicing good sleep hygiene can mitigate problems, so try to:

- Get daylight exposure every morning within thirty minutes to two hours of waking.
- Turn off screens two hours, or more, before bedtime.
- Stop any meals or snacks at least three hours before bedtime.
- Avoid strenuous exercise after dinner.
- Practice a wind-down routine.
- Sleep in a dark, cool room.
- Consider behavioral therapy for sleep.
- Lean in to sleep support supplements that include calming herbs and nutrients such as GABA, glycine, inositol, lemon balm, L-theanine, magnesium, and tryptophan.

out of the blue due to the fact that low hormones and the immune system activation and inflammatory processes that follow combine to override even the best sleep hygiene. Although the manifestation of sleep issues can vary widely from the frustration of being unable to fall asleep to the more concerning condition of sleep apnea whereby breathing repeatedly starts and stops throughout the night, untreated sleep loss is known to impact cognitive health and be a risk factor for dementia. For this reason, hormone restoration to reduce sleep disturbances is crucial.

At optimal levels, progesterone helps us fall asleep faster and enhances sleep quality via its positive effect on mood, anxiety, and depression. Estrogen's role in sleep has to do with its creation of serotonin and other neurotransmitters that affect melatonin, the hormone needed for sleep maintenance. Estrogen also keeps our body temperature low at night and has an antidepressant effect, both of which increase restful sleep. As sex hormones decline, sleep onset becomes delayed and both sleep duration and quality are diminished. For most women, initiating hormone replacement therapy to restore sex hormones to their optimal levels has substantial sleep benefits. In the absence of restoring sex hormones, incorporating strict sleep routines of avoiding bright lights and stimulatory activities along with using compounds such as cannabidiol (CBD) and cannabinol (CBN), and sleep support blends such as mentioned in the previous sidebar, can be very helpful.

STRESS: IT'S NOT GOING AWAY

Although we may not be able to reduce some of the stress in our lives, we can change the way we respond to stress by finding ways to mitigate and offset it. Understanding, too, that whether it's due to increased responsibilities during this life stage—from wearing many hats (childcare provider, partner role, caregiver to parents, household and career management)—or to declining sex hormones affecting quality of life through things like impaired sleep, midlife women tend to be stuck in a chronic state of stress. Over time, this existence destabilizes their ability to respond to stress because it "locks" the internal stress-handling machinery, called the autonomic nervous system, into always "seeing" and "responding to" stress.

The autonomic nervous system is made up of all our bodily systems working without any conscious input (such as digestion), as opposed to the somatic nervous system, which comprises all the functions over which we have conscious control (such as our motor functions). Within the autonomic nervous system are two branches: the sympathetic and the parasympathetic, each working respectively like the accelerator (threat response) and brake pedals (rest and relax response) on a car. For example, let's say you were walking through a crosswalk and suddenly hear a horn and see a car barreling toward you. In response to this, the sympathetic branch of your autonomic nervous system increases your heart rate and sends oxygen to your muscles so you can quickly jump out of the way. Once the car passes and you realize you are okay, the parasympathetic branch relaxes your muscles and returns your heart rate to normal. Just as with so many processes in the body, having a measured and balanced existence between these two branches is important for maintaining health.

For midlife women, all the stressors of this life phase can tip them over into being stuck in the sympathetic branch of the autonomic nervous system: always (mis)perceiving threats and waiting for and responding to the next one. This state of existence is catabolic (eroding) and, over time, can break down our bodies. If metabolic dysfunction and sleep disruption are also present, this sympathetic dominant pattern can increase risk by upregulating inflammation, blood sugar, and thyroid dysregulation. We cover more about the stress response and our adrenals in chapter 9.

Having a good set of tools for times of stress is essential for midlife women to remain healthy. A nightly glass of wine, staying up late and bingeing a show, or other forms of rumination are methods of avoidance, not stress relievers. Instead, whether prayer or meditation, breathing exercises or gratitude journaling, moderate exercise or rest, being in nature or whatever you choose, the modality does not matter provided it is restorative and involves positive choices. To be blunt: Life is stressful. Learning how to reframe it, looking for opportunities to manage it, and taking away any lessons learned are where growth happens . . . and if we women are capable of anything in this phase of life, it is the ability to adapt and persist!

MIDLIFE MOVEMENT: INSTEAD OF TAKING A WALK, YOU REALLY NEED THE GYM

As we discussed in chapter 5, maintaining mass and strength in muscles is crucial for mobility as well as metabolic health. Muscle mass in both men and women has been shown to decrease by 3 to 8 percent per decade after the age of thirty, and by 5 to 10 percent after age fifty. This loss of muscle mass includes reductions in both muscular strength (the ability of muscles to exert force, allowing us to lift objects) and muscular power (the ability to do work quickly, such as catching ourselves if we slip). These changes in muscle are known as *sarcopenia* and affect our ability to live independently. Although loss of muscle mass, strength, and power is part of the aging process, for women, the loss of estradiol accelerates these numbers. For this reason, movement in midlife needs to be thoughtfully directed at protecting muscle along with bone.

While there is a lot of messaging around walking, specifically getting 10,000 steps each day, unfortunately, studies have shown that walking is not enough to keep us operating independently. In fact, walking is less about muscle and bone and more about mood and stress mitigation. We are big fans of walking for a variety of reasons but do not use it as the tool to address muscle health: for that you need heavy things.

The decline in estradiol levels during and after the menopausal transition has detrimental effects on body composition, such as an increase in fat mass and a decrease in muscle mass, strength, and bone mineral density, all of which add up to an increases risk of frailty and chronic disease. Resistance, or strength, training has been shown to be particularly effective in counteracting most of the negative effects of the menopausal transition. In fact, strong evidence exists to show that progressive strength training in aging women has positive effects on lean body mass, muscle mass, strength, functional capacity, bone mass, and bone mineral density. Moreover, strength training reduces risks of falls and fractures and promotes physical and mental well-being, confidence, and happiness. In other words, while walking can be a lovely way to clear your mind and get out in nature, it is strength training that improves your health.

If you are new to exercise generally, or strength training specifically, we recommend first hiring a trained professional who can assess you for any range of motion limitations or other joint issues that may need accommodation, whether this is a physical therapist or personal trainer. The next step is to look at your nutrition (sufficient calories and protein intake) and sleep (adequate duration and quality) to make sure both are optimized for the proper fuel and energy needed with exercise. Finally, let your adrenal function (discussed in chapter 9) dictate the intensity and duration of your exercise. In other words, have your health foundations dialed in before signing up for that CrossFit, HIIT, boot camp, spin, or "body pump" class.

Once you decide you are ready to pursue movement that is built for midlife and beyond, invest in yourself by following a professionally designed plan or program. While pursuing a certain "aesthetic" is important for some, at the end of the day, we need a program designed to "move" us gradually to an improved state of strength and health. This means we

TEMPLATE FOR MIDLIFE MOVEMENT

Strength Training 3x/Week
- 10 minutes dynamic warm-up
- Compound exercises (squat, Romanian deadlift, push-up, lat pulldown)
- Coaching on form
- Choose heavy weights
- 5 to 8 reps for 3 sets

Moderate Intensity Cardio 1x/Week (Optional)
- Choose what you enjoy
- Keep heart rate at perceived level of 4 to 5 out of 10
- 30 to 45 minutes per session

Sprint Interval Training (SIT) 1x/Week (ONLY if Adrenals Are Healthy)
- Choose what you enjoy—and do it all-out
- Work/rest for 30 seconds/3 minutes or 8 seconds/12 seconds
- Repeat 4 to 8 times
- Perceived effort: 10 (work), 1 (rest)

Restorative Movement as Often as Possible
- Choose what you enjoy
- Dance, gentle yoga, casual walks, meditation

need to lift heavy things (strength training), push up our heart rate briefly (sprint intervals), and do some endurance work (sustained cardiometabolic output). If you have limited time to engage in formal exercise, prioritize strength training over anything else.

Don't despair, though. Being in the "gym" (whether at home or a public one) every day is not necessary and, in fact, would be counterproductive! Just as important as targeted movement in midlife is ample rest to recover from it. The body changes from exercise only when given time to adapt. So, pursuing other activities that are restorative is important, too. Finding the right mix does not have to be hard, so we prepared a template to help you keep things simple (see "Template for Midlife Movement" at left).

COMMUNITY: WHY YOU NEED YOUR "PACK"

For many women, midlife tends to be a slow shift into isolation. The decline in estradiol leads to a decline in oxytocin, a hormone produced in the brain that is essential for relationship building and maintenance, and this loss results in us not feeling as connected to others as before midlife. In addition, the physical and psychosocial changes as a result of declining hormones and their vast impacts across our brain and body can radically disrupt our self-image. On top of these changes, midlife women are often experiencing broader life changes, ranging from an empty nest and aging parents to career and relationship shifts. Because of this, midlife often brings feelings of shame and aloneness, which cause many to stop socializing, withdraw, and hibernate. The problem

is that humans are social creatures needing human interaction, so the absence of social connections can have profound effects on our overall health.

A lack of social connections can increase inflammation, blood pressure, incidence of heart disease, immune disorders, mental health disorders, and more. The good news is that creating and keeping strong social ties can lower stress and anxiety and help midlife women thrive. In fact, studies have shown that participation in formal social groups is associated with higher levels of physical activity and reduced severity of both physical and depressive symptoms during and after the menopausal transition.

As psychotherapist Esther Perel is known for saying, "The quality of our relationships determines the quality of our lives." Thus, whether it is joining a church, finding a community or hobby group, learning a new skill or sport, organizing a book or cooking club, or whatever brings you together with others and creates a sense of belonging, resist the urge to remove yourself from the world around you. While midlife brings about immense physical, emotional, and social changes, you can enjoy a fulfilling second chapter of life by investing in connection and finding your pack.

For many midlife women, investing in nutrition, gut health, sleep optimization, stress management, and a healthy mind-set is sufficient to stock their midlife toolbox to improve metabolic health. However, there are other support systems in the body that often suffer with sex hormone decline and, thus, may need some extra attention. Namely, women's adrenals, thyroid, and liver often struggle through this time of life. Thankfully, there are some nonmedical ways to support each of these and we will cover those next.

CHAPTER NINE

OTHER SUPPORT SYSTEMS THAT NEED ATTENTION IN MIDLIFE

UP TO THIS POINT, we have primarily focused on the role of the pituitary, ovaries, and sex hormones in women's health moving through the menopausal transition and beyond. Other organs and glands, some with their own hormones, also play a role in midlife health and, accordingly, need our attention, too. The most important of these body systems are the adrenal glands, thyroid gland, and liver. Understanding what they do, why they are relevant, and how to support them can help you transition through midlife in the healthiest way possible.

DO ADRENALS REALLY GET FATIGUED? NO.

The adrenal glands are two walnut-shaped glands that sit atop the kidneys. They are part of the hypothalamus-pituitary-adrenal (HPA) axis and are in charge of producing hormones that help regulate metabolism, immune system function, blood pressure, response to stress, and other essential functions. The primary hormones of the adrenal glands are cortisol, aldosterone, DHEA, and adrenaline.

During and after the menopausal transition, the adrenal glands secrete small amounts of sex hormones. This explains why a seventy-year-old woman with no ovarian function may still have detectable amounts of estrogen in her system. Although this is a good thing, the reality is that the amount of sex hormones secreted by the adrenal glands is not enough to support physiology and health as women age.

One of the most important roles the adrenal glands has is the way they modulate our response to stress. When the brain perceives something as stressful (whether mental or physical, real or perceived), a stress response is triggered in the HPA axis and the adrenals are called upon to release cortisol. As previously discussed, cortisol has various jobs but, in relation to stress, it causes an increase in your heart rate and blood pressure to provide a boost of energy to handle whatever the emergency is. After the initial stress is over, the system is designed to lower cortisol back to baseline until needed again.

The problem midlife women face is that, due to the physiologic impacts of declining sex hormones along with the realities of this stage of life, they often deal with multiple forms of stress and their nervous system becomes dominated by the "fight-or-flight" sympathetic branch of the autonomic nervous system. When cortisol is pumped out chronically, the brain slows cortisol production over time to protect the body. This is an adaptive mechanism with physiologic necessity because persistently high cortisol will break down the body. For example, having chronically high cortisol levels can lead to persistent high blood sugar (hyperglycemia), diabetes, inflammation, heart disease, lung problems, obesity, anxiety, depression, and more. In addition, if the body is constantly fighting stress, it will have a poor chance of fighting infections or other immune challenges; so, sometimes the brain's downregulation of cortisol is simply to enable a much needed immune response.

HPA AXIS DYSFUNCTION

The adaptive response of the brain to reduce cortisol production has been widely misunderstood and misrepresented. Too often, midlife women are told that if their cortisol level is low, they suffer from "adrenal fatigue." This term implies that "overuse" of the adrenal glands has resulted in a failure to produce stress hormones. The flaw in this logic is based on the idea that the adrenals control their production of hormones when, in fact, with the exception of Additon's disease which is an autoimmune process, they do not. Instead, hormones from the adrenals are under the direction of the brain as part of the HPA axis and their production does not fail due to overuse.

In addition to the flawed belief that adrenals fatigue and become unable to produce hormones, some claim that a chronic stress response will deplete other hormones, namely progesterone, due to a concept called the "pregnenolone steal." This theory posits that stress steals the mother hormone pregnenolone to make cortisol, which inevitably results in less pregnenolone to serve as a precursor for sex hormones. Again, there is no basis for this theory because it depends on there being some sort of "pool" of pregnenolone out of which all steroid hormones get made. In reality, it is well documented that hormone conversion from pregnenolone occurs in the mitochondria of each respective cell, not from a pool in the adrenals. Thus, just like "adrenal fatigue," a "pregnenolone steal" is not real.

While we reject these flawed theories, we absolutely do recognize the reality of what is called "HPA axis dysfunction." Within the HPA axis, three areas of the body work together to perform essential functions across multiple systems. None of them is independent, and each relies on the other (at least in some way, if not directly) to function properly. As long as things are going well, the system remains stable, but if an imbalance in one part develops, the other parts become dysfunctional.

HPA AXIS DYSFUNCTION

Extreme Fatigue

Insomnia

Trouble Coping with Stress

Brain Fog

Craving Sweet or Salty Foods

Digestive Problems

Weight Gain

Muscle and Joint Pain

How to Assess Your HPA Axis Health

Symptoms of HPA axis dysfunction include feeling wired but tired, having afternoon energy crashes, a lack of daytime hunger with nighttime snacking, low libido, muscle aches, forgetfulness and brain fog, poor multitasking, light sensitivity, and poor sleep quality. Common causes of HPA axis dysfunction range from trauma at an early age to chronic stress, overexercising, time zone travel, substance abuse, sleep deprivation, circadian rhythm mismanagement, poor nutrition, and exposure to environmental toxins. Because so many of the symptoms of HPA axis dysfunction overlap with low sex hormones, it is often difficult for midlife women to know what needs attention, so we recommend testing rather than guessing.

HPA axis function can be examined using something called the diurnal cortisol curve. Changes in cortisol levels from morning to evening should follow a distinct slope. By giving saliva or urine cortisol samples at various intervals during the day, your cortisol curve can be mapped and assessed. A healthy pattern has a robust morning response, with a gradual drop into the late afternoon, and a low point right before bed. Patterns in need of attention are those that are inverted, have spikes at night, or have no slope but, instead, are essentially flat—whether high or low. If any of these is the case, the risk of significant negative health outcomes is elevated.

How to Support Your HPA Axis Function

The most effective way to support optimal HPA axis function is by managing your habits and activities in alignment with the body's circadian rhythm, previously discussed. Getting morning sunlight, taking a walk outdoors, eating sufficient calories with optimal protein and fat, having broad mineral support with electrolytes, supplementing vitamins B and C (if needed), and incorporating stress management techniques, like breathing exercises and prayer or meditation, are all vital to keeping the system stable. By doing so, not only can you protect your metabolic health and mitigate some of the initial symptoms of declining hormones in midlife, but you can also maximize success should you choose to use hormone replacement therapy.

THYROPAUSE: IS YOUR THYROID SLOWING DOWN?

Unmanaged stress does not just affect the HPA axis and its hormones. Remember that the body is a system of systems, so if stress is chronically elevated and making demands of the hypothalamus and pituitary, disruption will also occur in the HPT axis regulating the thyroid. In addition to stress, the thyroid gland is, similar to the ovaries, also affected by aging. We refer to this as "thyropause."

Although thyroid problems can manifest as either too high (hyper) or too low (hypo) function, what midlife women experience most often in the menopausal transition is low function, with either a slowing of thyroid output or lower active thyroid hormone, or both. Regardless of the cause, without optimal circulating thyroid hormones, other hormones slow as well. For this reason, many symptoms of low thyroid overlap with symptoms of low sex hormones, such as fatigue, weight gain, rising cholesterol, heart palpitations, hair and skin

WIDE-RANGING EFFECTS OF THYROID HORMONE

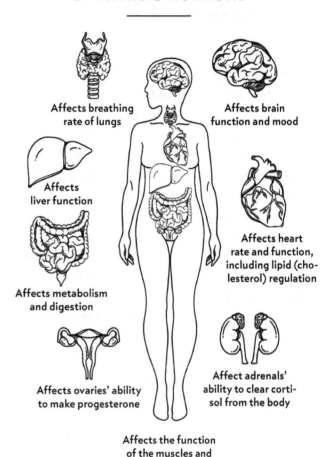

Affects breathing rate of lungs

Affects brain function and mood

Affects liver function

Affects heart rate and function, including lipid (cholesterol) regulation

Affects metabolism and digestion

Affect adrenals' ability to clear cortisol from the body

Affects ovaries' ability to make progesterone

Affects the function of the muscles and nerves of the eyes

changes, insomnia, mood and memory issues, constipation, and more.

While we absolutely need proper thyroid production via the HPT axis feedback loop, production is not the only issue. Because the primary hormone produced by the thyroid, thyroxine, or T4, is largely inactive, it must undergo an additional conversion step to become an active form, triiodothyronine, or

T3, to be utilized by the body, and this requires not only low stress and good gut health, but also optimal levels of important nutrients.

Conversion and Cofactors: Supporting Your Thyroid

Conversion of inactive thyroid hormone to its active form is uniquely sensitive to states of high inflammation as well as a disrupted microbiome. Optimizing your metabolic health and managing stress will help provide support to an aging thyroid, but certain vitamins and minerals are also required as cofactors, or helpers, for thyroid hormone production and conversion. Before any thyroid processes can begin, the body needs sufficient iodide, a salt-based form of the element iodine. Because iodine deficiency is a worldwide problem, supplementing with iodine is often recommended for thyroid support. The research on this, however, is incredibly controversial, so it is likely safer to simply ensure you are eating iodine-rich foods such as beef, liver, chicken, eggs, fish, and seaweed rather than taking an iodine supplement.

Thyroid hormones require additional nutrients as well, specifically copper, heme iron, selenium, tyrosine, vitamins A and B$_6$, and zinc. Provided you are eating a nutrient-dense whole foods diet that includes optimal animal protein, *and* that you have optimized your digestion and gut health, needing to supplement with these nutrients is unlikely with one exception—selenium. The thyroid gland requires the highest amount of selenium per gram of tissue compared to any other part of the body. Selenium is most often acquired via food—both animals and plants—but how much selenium is present in plant food often depends on the area from which it was sourced. In the United States, for example, the presence of selenium in the soil varies greatly from state to state, so someone in Michigan will get less selenium in local foods than someone in Colorado. Globally, the presence of selenium in soil differs greatly between and within countries due to geography (rocks and volcanic activities), climate variations (precipitation and aridity), and more.

Although some people may benefit from selenium supplementation, a more common issue with selenium is toxicity due to over-supplementing. Symptoms of selenium toxicity include foul, garlicky-smelling breath, whole body fatigue, gastrointestinal symptoms, lines that go side-to-side on fingernails, alopecia, and peripheral neuropathy. The tolerable upper limit of selenium supplementation is 400 mcg per day, but because it is often found in blended products like multivitamins, if you believe you need to supplement, it is important to check labels and take no more than 200 mcg daily from all supplements combined.

In addition to managing stress and getting optimal micronutrients for thyroid support, it is important to be mindful of other midlife changes that can affect the thyroid. For example, vitamin D deficiency, common in midlife, can impair thyroid function, as can blood sugar dysregulation, extended fasting or calorie restriction, certain medications, alcohol use, and smoking. Additionally, exposure to chemicals such as fluoride, nitrates, and pesticides has been shown to have a detrimental effect on thyroid health. For these reasons, we highly recommend considering a water filter if you do not know your water quality.

Finally, the majority of the process converting inactive T4 to active T3 comes from a process called deiodination, which takes place in our peripheral tissues, such as the liver and kidneys. For this reason, both a sluggish liver and chronic kidney disease are associated with impaired thyroid hormone conversion. The relationship of the liver to the thyroid is actually bidirectional: Not only can poor liver function impair thyroid hormone metabolism, but poor thyroid health can also compromise liver function. For this reason, liver health is a very important consideration in midlife and beyond.

OUR LIVERS ARE GETTING FAT AND WHY THIS MATTERS

The liver is a large, active, and very underappreciated organ. It sits in the upper-right abdomen under the rib cage and helps your body remove toxins, digest food, store energy, and make hormones. The liver's large size, fittingly, correlates with its critical role in the body: Anything consumed, whether food, alcohol, toxins, or medicine (including *any* type of hormone therapy), is filtered and detoxified by the liver. Your liver performs hundreds of jobs for you.

Unfortunately, due to a lifetime of poor dietary and lifestyle choices coupled with declining hormones, too many midlife women start the menopausal transition with poor liver health, despite a lack of symptoms. One liver condition that midlife women appear to have more than double the risk for compared to premenopausal women is "metabolic dysfunction-associated steatotic liver disease" (MASLD). Formerly referred to as "nonalcoholic fatty

liver disease," MASLD is classified by the accumulation of fat inside the liver of people who drink little to no alcohol, and is often coupled with obesity and dysregulated blood sugar, cholesterol and blood pressure. Other than from blood tests, early-stage MASLD is often undetectable but eventually leads to serious liver damage, including cirrhosis. If not addressed, all fatty liver diseases are associated with an increased risk of diabetes, cardiovascular disease, and cancer.

Because estrogen plays a role in blood sugar regulation, blood pressure, the distribution of body fat, and the uptake of free fatty acids from body tissues to the liver, it is believed that the loss of estrogen and its continued deprivation may explain the increased incidence of nonalcoholic fatty liver disease observed during and after the menopausal transition. For this reason, supporting liver function with healthy nutrition includes limiting the things that tax it the most—particularly alcohol.

HEALTHY HORMONES OR YOUR WEEKLY COCKTAIL: CHOOSE ONE

While regular alcohol consumption is most often equated with partying college students, sadly, research has found that, despite the potential health risks, many midlife women engage in what is referred to as "Mommy juice" culture—consuming alcohol daily, most often wine, and dismissing it as normal and acceptable as long as they appear respectable and in control. In addition, the media has put a health halo on the consumption of "moderate" drinking based on the flawed belief that "healthy" European cultures enjoy a daily glass of wine without consequence. In reality, there is nothing funny about the phrase "It's wine o'clock somewhere!" especially when it comes to the menopausal transition. Among other things, regular alcohol consumption raises the risk of breast cancer—a risk already increased with the loss of sex hormones—and, clearly, European women do not escape that reality given that breast cancer is the most frequently diagnosed cancer type in the World Health Organization's European Region.

Mix regular alcohol use with a high-carbohydrate/low-quality diet, lack of exercise, and high stress—all too common in midlife—and it should be no surprise that the liver suffers. As stated previously, one of the liver's important jobs is to detoxify hormones, whether we *make* them or *take* them. When this function is impaired due to alcohol consumption, we put ourselves at risk of disruption of hormone metabolism and detoxification, DNA damage, and cancer. What this means is that, as a midlife woman, if you are considering hormone therapy, you need to choose between your cocktail and your hormones. The association between the combination of hormone therapy and alcohol consumption with poor outcomes is so strong that we, unapologetically, caution midlife women against it—except for the very rare true special occasion.

HORMONE DETOX: LOVING YOUR LIVER

Whether you consume alcohol or not, sometimes even with good nutrition and lifestyle choices, the liver may need extra support to ensure it optimally performs one of its most important roles for midlife women: estrogen metabolism and detoxification.

The liver has two distinct phases through which it processes hormones: Phase 1 of liver detox is called hydroxylation, whereby enzymes are used to convert estrogens into one of three intermediate metabolites, each having a distinct effect on the body. These are:

- **2-hydroxyestrone (2-OH-E1):** This compound is considered the "least potentially harmful" to DNA due to its weak activity.

- **4-hydroxyestrone (4-OH-E1):** This compound is often referred to as "bad or potentially carcinogenic" because of its potential to harm DNA if not adequately detoxified in the body during in Phase 2 detoxification.

- **16-hydroxyestrone (16-OH-E1):** This compound is considered a strong proliferative agent in that it can stimulate tissue growth. This can be beneficial in terms of our bones but could be problematic in terms of our breasts; in other words, we need some 16-OH-E1, but not too much.

In Phase 2 of liver detoxification, estrogen gets neutralized and made water-soluble so you can pee or poop it out. The detoxification processes that occur in Phase 2 are called methylation, sulfation, and glucuronidation, with methylation being the most important because it reduces the potency of potentially carcinogenic compounds.

It is possible to determine how you detoxify your hormones by looking at these liver phases using a dried urine test analysis or 24-hour urine test, both of which can be ordered by consumers but need a health professional to interpret them. Ideally in Phase 1, liver detoxification results in an approximate breakdown of estrogen compounds into roughly 60 to 80 percent as 2-OH, 10 percent as 4-OH, and 10 to 30 percent as 16-OH, with strong neutralizing detoxification via the process of methylation in Phase 2. Sometimes these outcomes are influenced by genetics but, the good news is, you are not at the mercy of your genes. These pathways are malleable and can be improved with proper nutrition, targeted supplements, and healthy lifestyle choices.

As we stated, whether it is hormones you are still making or hormones you decide to take, healthy liver function is essential for midlife women. Avoiding alcohol, eating liver-loving nutrients, and optimizing nutrition and lifestyle habits can go a long way in protecting your health as you navigate the menopausal transition and beyond. Once you pull all the levers that are in your control, however, you may want to consider hormone therapy to ensure the extension of their important actions well beyond fertility and menstruation.

Because hormone therapy as a medical treatment for menopause has a confusing history and mixed reputation, we are going to devote the entire last part of this book to helping you sort through the topic so you can make your own informed opinion.

PART THREE

THE MISSING PIECE TO HEALTHY AGING

Restoring Hormones

MHT VS. HRT

What's the Difference and Does It Matter?

AS WE DISCUSSED BACK IN CHAPTER 2, the menopausal transition is much more than just a final menstrual cycle or the end of fertility. In fact, the term *menopause* is really just an arbitrary pseudo definition that is woefully inadequate. In reality, menopause speaks to the natural aging of the ovaries and the loss of the sex hormones produced by them. Because of this, menopause results in impaired physiologic processes and genetic signals throughout women's bodies and, as a result, leads to a negative shift in the potential healthspan of women. This is a process of variable duration and there is no finish line.

Despite the health concerns many women have or develop over menopause, the idea of hormone therapy to address those concerns can be very polarizing. Whether you are curious about hormone therapy or believe it is dangerous and not an option for you, the next chapters address much of the misinformation that exists on this topic and we urge you to read them, regardless of your interest, beliefs, or fears.

UNDERSTANDING THE IMPLIED MESSAGING IN DIFFERENT TERMS

When menopause is viewed narrowly as simply the loss of menstruation and fertility, attention is paid only to the transient symptoms that may or may not accompany this loss. When menopause is viewed as a catalyst for declining healthspan, attention is paid to the larger effects on one's overall health and symptoms.

Two different views of what menopause entails and means for women's health also results in different terms being used when talking about hormone therapy. This distinction is most visible when the term *MHT*, or *menopausal hormone therapy*, is used versus the term *HRT*, or *hormone replacement therapy*. To be clear, for the vast majority of women, the terms simply refer to the use of hormones after menopause and, accordingly, to many women they are interchangeable with other terms, such as *HT*, or *hormone therapy*, or even *BHRT*, or *bioidentical hormone replacement therapy* (more on this in the next chapter). When it comes to medical providers and researchers, however, the difference between MHT and HRT comes down to treatment goals.

WHY TERMINOLOGY MATTERS

MHT uses short-term, low doses of estrogen, either alone or with progesterone, to manage menopausal symptoms such as hot flashes, dry vaginal tissue, and osteoporosis. On the other hand, HRT replaces sex hormones to premenopausal levels.

So, unlike HRT, *MHT is not about physiologic replacement or trying to deal with health issues—its only aim is symptom suppression.* To that end, if a woman does not have a uterus, she will not be given progesterone with MHT because providers not focused on using hormone therapy as whole body health supportive (mistakenly) fail to see progesterone as having any impact on women's health beyond protecting her uterus. This is flawed thinking. As we describe in chapter 3, progesterone acts well outside the uterus and works *with* estrogen, not just in opposition to it. The biggest problem with the thinking behind MHT is that it takes less estrogen to suppress a hot flash than it does to maintain overall brain health, cardiovascular health, and bone health, not to mention all the other processes affected by the loss of sex hormones.

Research is showing that women need physiologic levels, or those levels prior to menopause, along with rhythms of sex hormones, to preserve their health and mitigate the effects of aging. The conventional

PREMATURE MENOPAUSE

FOR SOME PROVIDERS, HRT refers to replacing lost hormones due to premature menopause in instances such as surgical removal of the ovaries, premature ovarian insufficiency, or chemotherapy-induced ovarian failure. What this means is that some providers use HRT to refer to "unnatural" menopause treatment and MHT to refer to "natural" menopause treatment. The irony is that one choice (the former) recognizes the importance of sex hormones for a *younger* woman's health and the other (the latter) ignores that relevance for *older* women. In addition, another term used frequently today, *BHRT*, or *bioidentical hormone replacement therapy*, refers to the use of natural hormones versus synthetic hormones.

medical world is seemingly not only stuck on the "smallest dose for the shortest amount of time" mind-set, but also on the view that *only* symptomatic women should receive hormones. This is why it is so important for women to know and understand the difference between the implied meanings of MHT and HRT. By understanding this difference, you can identify which health care providers are the best choice to help you optimize your health and quality of life rather than merely stopping your symptoms and complaints.

WHATEVER YOU CALL IT, IT'S NOT JUST ONE THING

It would be easy to think, then, that any health care provider favoring HRT should have the right approach. Unfortunately, it is not that easy. A woman's long-term health is not just about having *any* estrogen but rather about having the right types or forms, the right mode of delivery, the right levels, and the right rhythms or cycles. Although use of the term HRT speaks to the objective for treatment, it does not reveal the method that will be used. HRT is not a single, off-the-shelf, uniform commercial product, and, even more important, what is proper for one woman is often different from what is necessary for another. The good news is, in chapter 12, we provide a road map to navigate the many types of hormone therapies available. Before we get to that, however, we want you to have a deep understanding of the history of hormone therapy.

HISTORICAL USE OF MEDICAL HORMONE THERAPIES

The use of hormones as medical therapy is not new; it is, in fact, centuries old! Around 200 BCE, Chinese practitioners isolated sex and pituitary hormones from human urine and used them for a multitude of medicinal purposes. In the 600s CE, Sun Simiao first administered the glandular extracts of deer and sheep thyroid to human patients with an enlarged thyroid (goiter) and achieved a variety of benefits. By 1025 CE, Chinese medicine practitioners used extracts of female urine to treat menstrual and other female problems.

The use of hormone extracts continued to be explored, and by 1855 European researchers were studying endocrine glands and the hormones they secreted. In 1872, Robert Battey pioneered the "ovariotomy" whereby (diseased) ovaries were removed from women who were experiencing "menstrual madness" (today referred to as premenstrual dysphoric disorder, or PMDD) as well as dysmenorrhea and bleeding from uterine tumors. When these women subsequently developed hot flashes and vaginal atrophy, it was hypothesized that the ovaries make a substance that the absence of which causes various symptoms. In 1896, after observing that "oöphorectomy" (removal of ovaries) in cows prolonged their lactation time, Sir George Beatson wrote a paper that demonstrated that removing the ovaries to cut off estrogen caused regression of breast cancer in women. By 1897, Hubert Fosbery was using extracts from cow ovarian tissue to treat hot flashes and other menopausal symptoms in women and concluding that menstruation was related to ovulation.

NATURAL ESTROGEN'S DISCOVERY AND EARLY CLINICAL APPLICATIONS

Shortly after Fosbery's discovery, various labs in Europe extracted estrogen from the urine of pregnant women, which then led to the development of estrogen products. In 1923, three key investigators, Edgar Allen, Edward Doisy, and Adolf Butenandt, managed to purify estrogen by studying follicular fluid from female hogs. In 1929, Fuller Albright expanded upon the use of biological material to create crystallized estrogen and, over the subsequent years, engaged in significant research that proved many clinical benefits of estrogen, showing its supportive role in preserving bone and heart health as well as its ability to block hot flashes and prevent ovulation.

In the 1930s, a Canadian researcher extracted estrogen from the placentas and urine of pregnant women and the result was Emmenin, the first commercial estrogen product, marketed by the pharmaceutical company Ayerst. Because it came from pregnant women, this product contained the primary estrogen of pregnancy, estriol. Then, in 1949, Russell Marker discovered that a specific Mexican yam with the highest level of diosgenin, a plant steroid molecule, could be used to synthesize progesterone, and this led to research that showed ovulation could be blocked using progesterone. Ultimately, these discoveries led to the development of the first birth control pill in 1960 and substantially changed the role of women in society and the workplace.

SYNTHETIC ESTROGEN AND THE COMMERCIALIZATION OF HORMONES

Because Emmenin was expensive to produce due to its human sourcing, in 1942, Ayerst introduced Premarin, a synthetic estrogen, as its replacement, with the goal of creating a market for treating hot flashes and other menopausal symptoms. Premarin is a complex mix of more than fifty different estrogens derived from the urine of pregnant horses (also called conjugated equine estrogen, or CEE). After a corporate merger, the company became Wyeth and received approval by the US Food and Drug Administration (FDA) to bring Premarin to market for human use. Around the same time, other companies were exploring additional forms of synthetic estrogen given to women via patches, pills, and injections, all approved by the FDA.

Shortly thereafter, because of research from Europe showing how estrogen blocked ovulation, a new use was discovered for synthetic estrogen beyond menopause. The result was FDA approval in 1957 of a product called Enovid to treat menstrual disorders. By 1960, Enovid, a combination of synthetic estrogen and synthetic progesterone, was approved for use as a contraceptive, enabling women to engage in sex without fearing pregnancy. Of note, despite these being very new and novel therapies at the time, other than experimenting with Enovid on Puerto Rican women, no studies were done on the safety or effectiveness of synthetic estrogen.

As the use of synthetic estrogen therapies for "menopausal disorders" started to gain traction, a New York City–based British gynecologist, Dr. Robert Wilson, wrote a book called *Feminine Forever*. In it,

Wilson argued that "untreated" menopause robbed women of their femininity and ruined the quality of their lives, and that menopause was a hormone-deficiency disease curable and preventable by taking estrogen. He referred to estrogen therapy as a biological revolution and asserted that "estrogen does not change a woman, it keeps her from changing." This book was paradoxically both widely embraced as shining a light on menopause being a time to redefine women's health, and resoundingly rejected as it promoted notions that aging is pathological. Either way it was viewed, *Feminine Forever* was instrumental in framing estrogen therapy as a logical consideration to address menopause. Despite delivering some persuasive ideas, Wilson was later discredited when it was discovered he was being paid by pharmaceutical companies making estrogen.

Given all the attention in the media, medical circles, and scientific publications, synthetic hormone products proliferated and led to a steady increase in the use of synthetic hormone therapy to address "menopausal disorders," eventually doubling and tripling by 1970. Accordingly, the market for drug companies and physicians to increase prescriptions of synthetic estrogen formulations exploded and, by 1975, estrogen was the fifth most prescribed drug in the United States.

HINTS OF PROBLEMS: CANCER, BLOOD CLOTS, AND CARDIOVASCULAR DISEASE

Around 1975, a short study indicated that unopposed estrogen supplements in any form were associated with an increased risk of endometrial cancer. As a result, many doctors discouraged hormone therapy use. However, that study also gave rise to another, which revealed that reducing the dosage of oral estrogen and combining it with progestin, a synthetic form of progesterone, could reduce any endometrial cancer risk. Henceforth, estrogen plus a progestin was referred to as "combined therapy" and recommended for women with an intact uterus. Not surprisingly, hormone therapy for menopause treatment was, once again, met with renewed enthusiasm.

Simultaneous with these cancer concerns, Great Britain reported an alarming number of healthy young women suffering from blood clots after starting hormone therapy with a form of Enovid. The British government was so concerned that it phased out of circulation all high-dose synthetic estrogen pills associated with these clots. Despite similar reports of clots in the United States, the pills continued to be available to women while researchers pursued long-term follow-up studies. Because they felt that women with strong medical knowledge would be the best subjects, they focused on synthetic estrogen pill use by nurses, leading to the Nurses' Health Study.

Begun in 1976, the Nurses' Health Study was an uncontrolled observational study in which women completed complex questionnaires every two years over a period of several years. The study had different parts with different conclusions. One part looked at women taking oral contraceptives and revealed a higher risk of stroke, heart disease, and breast cancer while on birth control that disappeared once the pills were stopped. Another part looked at postmenopausal women and concluded that recently postmenopausal women using hormone therapy enjoyed both a reduced risk of developing heart disease as well as a lower risk of dying from heart disease (although women long past menopause with existing heart disease received no such benefits). Because the study ignored impacts from family disease history, shift work, alcohol use, toxin exposure, sedentary versus active lifestyles, body mass index (BMI) scores, and more, it did receive some criticism; however, due to wide public trust at that time in the FDA and government agencies, generally, the idea of using hormones to prevent the chronic diseases of aging started to take root.

Additional early studies convincingly showed hormone therapy could relieve women of menopause symptoms such as hot flashes and weight gain as well as prevent osteoporosis and heart disease. Because population data clearly showed that, before meno-pause, women had less heart disease than men, but after menopause, women's incidence of heart disease caught up to that of men, the conclusions around hormone therapy and disease risk became incredibly compelling. In fact, hormone therapy became so well accepted that it was ultimately endorsed by the American Heart Association, the American College of Physicians, and the American College of Obstetricians and Gynecologists as a *preventive therapy for the chronic diseases of menopausal women.*

Heart Disease Fears Renewed

By the late 1980s, despite the enthusiasm around using hormone therapy to address disease risk in menopause, an international group of scientists raised concerns about potential negative effects from synthetic progesterone (progestins) on the cardiovascular system. These experts' claims were compelling enough to cause the FDA to require randomized clinical trials to demonstrate any claims of hormone therapy–induced cardiovascular benefits. Five major trials followed over the next decade.

The HERS trials consisted of a two-part study with the goal of assessing the safety of Premarin with Provera (a synthetic progestin) for the prevention of recurrent coronary heart disease in women *with known atherosclerosis.* The first part of the HERS trials showed that these women had a slight increase of disease in year one of their hormone therapy but that the disease regressed in years three to five. The second part of the study showed that the regression disappeared over time—*essentially contradicting the Nurses' Health Study.* Unfortunately, although the trial was looking at a certain subset of women (those with coronary plaques), its conclusions were applied to all women.

Researchers felt strongly that estrogen and progestin conferred benefit to women's hearts, so they conducted another trial over three years using different combinations of Premarin and Provera—the Postmenopausal Estrogen/Progestin Interventions Study (PEPI). Using robust study design parameters, the data showed *favorable effects on LDL (bad) cholesterol and fibrinogen,* both suspected to play a significant role in heart disease, but *no effects on blood pressure in healthy postmenopausal women.*

Shortly after the PEPI results were published, researchers began a sister-pair of rigorous trials. Both the Estrogen in the Prevention of Atherosclerosis Trial (EPAT) and the Women's Estrogen-Progestin Lipid-Lowering Hormone Atherosclerosis Regression Trial (WELL-HART) were designed to determine the effects of hormone therapy on atherosclerosis progression in postmenopausal women with and without preexisting clinical vascular disease. These important studies showed that *initiation of hormone therapy early in postmenopausal women who had no vascular disease maintained vascular health and reduced vascular aging and progression of atherosclerosis, while the effect was neutral for women with preexisting vascular disease.*

Almost simultaneous with these studies, British researchers launched The Million Women Study, which looked at the effects of hormone therapy on breast cancer. Like the Nurses' Health Study, this was an uncontrolled observational study that relied on questionnaires completed by participants using either no hormone therapy, estrogen-only therapy, or estrogen plus synthetic progestin hormone therapy. It concluded that, in comparison to women using no hormones at all, hormone therapy created a twofold increase in breast cancer in women using combined therapy and a 1.3 times increase in women using estrogen-only therapy.

At the time, the combined effect of these major studies was that, despite decades of research, no consensus could be reached establishing public policy guidance on the safety of hormone therapy. There was no question, however, that among postmenopausal women, heart disease, cancer, and osteoporosis were driving poor health outcomes, and that heart disease and cancer were the leading causes of death for these women. The only agreement to be found was that more testing via clinical trials was needed. Unfortunately, because of the vested interest of the pharmaceutical companies whose products were the subject of past studies, no attention was given to the fact that despite the availability of natural hormones, only synthetic hormones were being used in menopausal women. For this reason, the most influential study to come was focused entirely on proving the benefits of *synthetic* hormones.

As you will see in the next chapter, the study and outcome of synthetic hormones were used as a basis to deny hormone therapy to millions of women, and this extrapolation of poor hormone therapy to characterize all hormone therapy turned out to be an incredible disservice to women's health.

CHAPTER ELEVEN

HORMONE THERAPY

Why You Might Fear It and Why You Shouldn't

IF HORMONES ARE SO IMPORTANT, why the controversy over hormone therapy?

As we demonstrated in part 1, it is without dispute that women's sex hormones play a critical role in their overall whole body health. Despite this reality, most women have been taught to fear them, including even our own doctors. Why? Sadly, today's modern view of hormones for women in middle age and beyond is largely the result of a single study born out of the absence of public policy due to inconsistent scientific research coupled with initiatives by pharmaceutical companies to create a market for women's hormone care. Enter the Women's Health Initiative, or WHI.

UNDERSTANDING STUDY DESIGNS

We are going to review various studies on hormone therapy here and because there are, literally, thousands of ways to design a study, some have more reliability in their outcomes than others. We could devote an entire chapter explaining all the relevant aspects of study methods and design but, instead, we are going to give you a condensed, quick guide to the most important terms you need to know to navigate the field of health research.

The most important thing to know is that much of health research—especially the kind that gets "clicks" and makes headlines—can be broken down into two basic types: observational and interventional.

- **Observational/Correlational/Epidemiological:** Scientists observe and gather data and descriptive information on habits, beliefs, or events in a specified population, but do not influence or intervene in any way.

- **Interventional/Experimental:** Scientists do intervene, such as provide study subjects a drug or perform an operation on them, or at least use statistical methods to mimic intervention.

Then, within these types of studies, different approaches and factors can either increase or decrease the study's strength:

- **Active Treatment vs. Placebo-Controlled:** All participants receive treatment vs. two groups existing with one receiving treatment and the other receiving a placebo.

- **Cohort vs. Multi-Arm:** A predefined group of people who are observed and followed over time vs. studying two different populations receiving a specified treatment; having multiple arms allow the effects of different interventions to be compared in a single study.

- **Control vs. Experimental:** Study subjects who do not have the disease, treatment, or outcome vs. those who do.

- **Longitudinal vs. Cross-Sectional:** Correlational research that repeatedly examines the same individuals to detect any changes that might occur over a period of time vs. different samples (or a cross-section) of the population at one point in time.

- **Open vs. Blind/Double-Blind Trial:** When both the researchers and participants know which treatment is being administered vs. when neither the researchers nor the participants know which participants are in the control group or the experimental group.

- **Prospective vs. Retrospective:** A study that moves forward in time, or for which the outcomes are being observed as they occur, vs. a study that collects historical data and looks back on outcomes that have already taken place.

- **Randomized Control vs. Case Control:** Treatment groups are comparable with the only difference between them being the intervention (as in, whether they received the drug or not), so any difference in outcome between the two groups can be attributed to the intervention vs. two existing groups differing in outcome being identified and compared on the basis of some supposed causal attribute.

- **Single vs. Multicenter:** A trial conducted according to a single protocol and at a single site vs. a trial conducted according to a single protocol but at different locations, and conducted by various researchers, thereby providing a larger sample size.

The "gold standard" for health research are studies that are interventional, randomized, double-blind, placebo-controlled studies; however, they can be costly, time-consuming, and complex to design, implement, and monitor. Because of this, many studies exist that do not adhere to these standards. This does not mean that the non–gold standard studies are without merit, but it does require some understanding of what limitations and confounding factors may affect their outcomes and the strength of their conclusions.

THE NUTS AND BOLTS OF THE WOMEN'S HEALTH INITIATIVE

Started in 1998, the enormous United States–based $725 million Women's Health Initiative, or WHI, had three parts—a clinical trial, an observational study, and a community prevention study. The trial portion was the largest randomized study to date aimed at evaluating the effect of hormone therapy on the most common causes of death and disability in postmenopausal women, such as cardiovascular disease, cancer, and osteoporosis. Sponsored by the National Institutes of Health (NIH), it was intended to last eight years and resolve the controversy over whether menopause should be embraced as a natural life transition, a position taken by the feminist movement at the time, or, as proposed by others, viewed as a hormone deficiency that is totally preventable with hormone therapy.

The WHI clinical trial had two arms, one using women who had an intact uterus and who were given either a placebo *or* conjugated equine estrogen with a progestin (CEE, a.k.a. Premarin, with medroxyprogesterone acetate, or MPA, a combination called PremPro), and the other with women who had no uterus and were given either a placebo *or* only conjugated equine estrogen (CEE). With the first arm, in 2002, after only 5.6 years of follow-up, early preliminary results appeared to show an increased incidence of both coronary heart disease and breast cancer. Accordingly, despite also showing reductions of osteoporotic fractures and colon cancer, this arm of the trial was immediately discontinued.

With the second arm, in 2004, after 6.8 years of follow-up, early results showed a small increased risk of ischemic stroke (blood clot) and, despite also showing a reduction of osteoporotic fractures and colon cancer as well as no increase in risk of breast cancer or cardiovascular disease, this arm was also prematurely discontinued. From these results, it was "concluded" that estrogen was inherently dangerous: Not only did it "cause" cancer but it also increased the risk for heart disease, stroke, blood clots, and dementia. Instantly, the overall message on HRT turned incredibly negative.

Good Intentions Gone Wrong

The abrupt stoppage of the WHI clinical trial attracted enormous media attention and the result was widespread panic. Of the approximately sixteen million US women using hormone therapy at the time, more than 80 percent stopped it immediately, with most believing that what had been prescribed by their doctor to keep them healthy was actually "deadly." Likewise, doctors refused to prescribe hormone therapy to menopausal women, telling them to just put up with their hot flashes.

Following suit, governments in the United States, United Kingdom, and Australia joined the chorus of doom with respect to hormone therapy and immediately issued new guidelines, stating that the only reason women and their doctors should consider hormone therapy would be for treatment of "moderate to severe" hot flashes or significant risk of osteoporosis fracture. Even under those circumstances, it was decided that hormone therapy was to be used only at the lowest possible dose and for the shortest amount of time and definitely *not* for chronic disease prevention in postmenopausal women. Twenty years later, prominent warnings and limitations on use of hormone therapy remain.

Due to the governments' positions, the drug companies were also throttled into disavowing hormone therapy. Wyeth, the maker of Premarin, faced thousands of lawsuits over its formulations (paying more than $330 million to resolve claims) and ultimately was sold to Pfizer in 2009. The final straw in this panic cascade was that doctors and medical schools caved, too, so that to this day, the crucial information about the role of hormones in women's whole body health, let alone the difference between equine and bioidentical hormones, is not taught to students. The result? Multiple generations of general practitioners, endocrinologists, and gynecologists too scared to prescribe hormone therapy, and another generation or two thoroughly lacking the knowledge, confidence, and experience to do so.

HORMONE THERAPY GETS A SECOND CHANCE: RECONSIDERING THE WOMEN'S HEALTH INITIATIVE

Thankfully, despite the rash actions initially taken after the Women's Health Initiative (WHI) was stopped, the original investigators as well as other researchers continued for decades to review follow-up results, eventually offering clarifications for their initial conclusions. What they admitted was that the "risks" for certain safety aspects were overestimated and that when hormone therapy is initiated in the fifty to fifty-nine age range or for those less than ten years postmenopause, there is actually a lower risk of death from heart disease, a lower risk of death from any cause, and no increased risk from stroke. Despite the study authors' attempts to clarify their findings, a deeper dive into the details of the WHI looks at the subjects studied, the interventions used, and the design parameters—and this is where the flaws become glaringly obvious.

The first issue with the WHI is that they used the wrong subjects. Despite the average age of menopause in the United States being fifty-one years old, the average age of WHI subjects was sixty-three years old (160,000 women aged fifty-nine to seventy-nine), meaning many of these women were more than a decade past their last menstrual cycle and had already experienced declines in vascular health due to age-related changes, putting them at greater risk for cardiovascular events. In addition to being too old, the WHI women were not metabolically healthy, as many were obese, prediabetic, and smokers who had very poor diet and lifestyle habits.

In fact, more than 25 percent were already on statins before joining the study. In addition, the WHI women were not prescreened for cancer, heart disease, or osteoporosis. Finally, WHI women with symptoms such as hot flashes were excluded from the study because researchers feared that if these women were randomly placed in the placebo group, they would stop the placebo and drop out of the trial entirely.

The second biggest problem with the WHI details involved the hormones used. The physiologic changes that result from menopause are due to the loss of *estradiol* and *progesterone*. The WHI's "hormones" consisted of Premarin as estradiol and Provera as progesterone. Premarin is derived from horse urine and, as such, is an animal, not human, waste product that has already been processed through the liver and excreted. Because of it being a downstream metabolite of a horse's estrogen, it contains ten *known* estrogens, with more not known, the majority being estrone and almost no estradiol. Since estrone stimulates only one of the main estradiol receptors in the female body, it creates an unnatural and imbalanced effect.

The third biggest problem with the WHI was the way the hormones were administered. The Premarin (fake estradiol) was taken as an estrogen pill, which means it was being absorbed in the intestines with a "first pass" through the liver. When estrogens are taken orally, the production of many clotting factors increases, which leads to a higher incidence of stroke—as seen in both arms of the study. In addition, the WHI women were given hormones in a static fashion, meaning in the same amount every day. As was explained in chapter 2, a woman's natural menstrual cycle has a rhythm with different hormones fluctuating at different times; beyond just causing a monthly bleed, this rhythm is biologically relevant because it controls genetic signals for physiologic actions throughout the female body.

Finally, the WHI used the wrong math. The WHI researchers negligently misportrayed *statistical* risk

THE MOST PROMINENT CONCLUSIONS *walked back* by WHI investigators include:

- **Hormone therapy increases the risk of breast cancer**
  - » After almost twenty years of follow-up, they now report that estrogen actually decreases the risk of breast cancer, decreases the risk of death from it, and decreases the risk of death from all causes.

- **Hormone therapy did not have a clinically meaningful effect on health-related quality of life for women in menopause**
  - » They now admit that hormone therapy is the most effective treatment for managing menopausal hot flashes and improves women's quality of life.

- **Hormone therapy increases the risk of cardiac events, strokes, and cognitive decline as well as all-cause mortality**
  - » They have rescinded every one of those, especially when hormone therapy is initiated within ten years of a woman's final menstrual period.

in order to claim *clinical* risk by using language such as "almost reached nominal statistical relevance." Despite the broad risk claims made, out of ten thousand person-years in the WHI, there were only seven more cardiac events, eight more strokes, eight more pulmonary emboli, and eight more breast cancers than in placebo users. Even worse, the WHI researchers actually ignored their own data. Subsequent analysis of the results showed that for the WHI women who took estrogen only (those without a uterus), 44 percent actually had a *reduced incidence* of breast cancer than women who took no estrogen at all. Even more persuasive, results also clearly showed that for WHI women in their fifties (about 10 percent of the subjects), even with the oral synthetic forms and continuous regimen of hormone therapy there was a 30 percent *decrease* in all-cause mortality.

All told, the WHI researchers designed a study with the aim of evaluating the role of hormone therapy in menopause *as a preventive therapy to protect cardiovascular and bone health* and yet chose to study already unhealthy, older women as their subjects; gave them a dangerous combination of fake chemical or animal-derived hormones in a nonphysiologic manner that created health risks; and then misconstrued the data and applied sweeping conclusions to all women as well as to all forms, types, combinations, dosing, and patterns of hormones, including even hormones that mimic *human* hormones.

As one of our mentors likes to say, the WHI was the crazy equivalent of doing a study with children eating raspberry-flavored jelly beans, finding an increase in cavities, diabetes, and obesity, and declaring that no one should ever eat an organic raspberry.

DAMAGE DONE . . . *BUT* HOPE ON THE HORIZON?

Basically, the WHI left women throughout the world without an effective option to preserve their health for the past twenty-plus years. A recent study showed that women who discontinued their hormone therapy because of the WHI, despite remaining physically active, lost bone mass whereas women who continued their therapy maintained their bones. Another analysis examined the mortality toll on women aged fifty to fifty-nine who were not given HRT following publication of the WHI's "findings" and showed that between 2002 and 2011, a minimum of 18,601, and as many as 91,610, excess deaths occurred among these women, with the actual toll of excess mortality likely between 40,292 and 48,835. Add to this the statistics we shared in chapter 1 that, in the United States alone, menopause costs $1.8 billion in lost work time per year and $26.6 billion annually when medical expenses are added. Given these human and financial costs, it is critical that the WHI narrative be put to rest.

POST–WOMEN'S HEALTH INITIATIVE SCIENCE AND PRACTICE

Thankfully, despite horrible messaging takeaways for women, doctors, government agencies, medical schools, and more that hormones, generally, are dangerous—even our own natural hormones —dogged scientific researchers have continued to study hormone therapy. Their work has consolidated the view that hormones are actually highly beneficial when given to women at the right time in the right forms (we summarize these studies for you following). In fact, huge amounts of randomized trial data combined with results from observational studies, animal studies, historical interventions, and basic science show that when started within a decade of menopause, proper hormone therapy either protects from or has a null effect on women's risk of:

- All-cause mortality
- Atherosclerosis
- Cancer
- Cardiovascular disease
- Cognitive decline
- Diabetes
- Genitourinary syndrome
- Osteoporosis
- Stroke

   To put it more bluntly, from a scientific perspective, ample well-designed studies have shown systemic hormone therapy to be an absolutely valid sex-specific and time-dependent primary preventive therapy for women's whole body health.

Better Trials, Better Evidence

The following studies were better designed and resulted in better evidence-based outcomes.

E3N: FRENCH PROSPECTIVE COHORT STUDY

This study was initiated in 1990 to test hypotheses related to the relationship between hormone therapy and cancer, as well as diet and cancer.

- Data from more than eighty thousand female teachers between the ages of forty and sixty-five were used.

- The study participants completed questionnaires every two to three years that asked about dietary habits and general lifestyle characteristics as well as medical events.

- Various hormone therapies were utilized by 70 percent of the women for an average of seven years.

- Results showed that estrogen, when combined with progesterone, resulted in zero increased risk of breast cancer, whereas estrogen used alone or with a progestin showed a significantly increased risk.

- The study also showed that smoking, high body mass index, alcohol consumption, sedentary living, and low fiber intake all increased the risk of breast and lung cancers, diabetes, and asthma in midlife women.

THE KRONOS EARLY ESTROGEN PREVENTION STUDY (KEEPS)

This randomized, double-blind, placebo-controlled trial began in 2005 shortly after WHI stopped and ran through 2009 with the goal of examining the effects of different hormone therapies on cardiovascular disease, specifically progression of carotid artery thickness and arterial plaque changes.

- The trial was a multicenter, five-year trial studying women aged forty-two to fifty-eight who had completed menopause within the prior three years.

- The hormone therapy used was either low-dose conjugated equine estrogen daily with twelve days of oral progesterone or weekly doses of transdermal estradiol with twelve days of progesterone or placebo.

- Both forms of estrogen were in doses lower than what was used in the WHI due to clotting concerns.

- After four years, despite showing benefit to cardiovascular disease risk, the researchers claimed their results supported the use of both forms of hormone therapy based on the fact that topical estradiol therapy improved sexual function and no adverse events were reported from either form of therapy.*

THE DANISH OSTEOPOROSIS PREVENTION STUDY (DOPS)

This study, published in 2012, was a twenty-year partly randomized trial to evaluate whether hormone therapy started shortly after menopause reduced the risk of later osteoporotic fractures.

- This trial involved more than one thousand women who were treated early in menopause with estradiol and a progestin, or with estradiol alone if they had no uterus.

- The study reported a significantly decreased risk of heart failure and myocardial infarction (heart attack) when hormone therapy was started within ten years after menopause.

- Women given estradiol without a progestin also had a significant reduction in breast cancer incidences.

MILLION WOMEN STUDY REANALYSIS

Published in 2012, this study debunked the original study conclusions that previously causally linked hormone therapy to breast cancer.

* REANALYSES OF KEEPS SHOWED that because the conjugated equine estrogen used was at a much lower dose of estrogen than had been used in previous trials, its safety could not be validated by KEEPS because the level was nearly insignificant. Additionally, the transdermal estradiol dose was too low to get adequate estradiol into the blood and confer any benefits. Accordingly, the original conclusions that oral CEE is safe and that transdermal estradiol does not benefit cardiovascular health could not be supported because neither dose was high enough to evaluate properly.

- This reanalysis showed no causal relationship between hormone therapy and breast cancer.

- The data also demonstrated no increased risk of blood clots with use of transdermal estradiol.

EARLY VS. LATE INTERVENTION TRIAL WITH ESTRADIOL (ELITE)

Published in 2015, ELITE was a single-center, randomized, double-blind, placebo-controlled trial of healthy postmenopausal women (either no menses for more than six months or surgically induced). Its focus was to test a hypothesis that hormone therapy confers greater benefits when initiated earlier rather than later after menopause.

- Participants were screened for diabetes and coronary artery deposits of plaque and heart disease.

- The study results showed that estradiol—with or without progesterone—was protective against atherosclerosis when initiated less than six years postmenopause but had a neutral effect when initiated more than ten years postmenopause.

FINNISH STUDY

Published in 2016, this was a large observational study of 489,105 women using hormone therapy between 1994 and 2009. Its focus was to compare breast cancer mortality rates between users and nonusers of hormone therapy.

- This study showed that the risk of dying from breast cancer was significantly reduced in all users of hormone therapy, regardless of duration of use, age, or whether the hormone therapy was estrogen only or estrogen plus progestin.

- The big conclusion was that the age at hormone therapy initiation showed no association with breast cancer mortality.

ANCILLARY STUDY OF KEEPS ON FEMALE SEXUAL FUNCTION

This study, released in 2017, was a four-year prospective, randomized, double-blind, placebo-controlled trial of menopausal hormone therapy in healthy, recently menopausal women. Its focus was to examine the effects of transdermal or oral estrogen therapy on sexual function in recently postmenopausal women over time.

- Women were randomized to receive oral conjugated equine estrogen, transdermal estradiol, or a placebo.

- The study showed that transdermal estradiol resulted in a significant yet moderate improvement in female sexual function compared to both oral conjugated equine estrogen and the placebo.
  - Specifically, transdermal estradiol was associated with a significant increase in lubrication and decreased pain.

REPLENISH TRIAL: THE BIRTH OF BIJUVA

This 2018 FDA Phase 3, twelve-month, randomized, double-blind, placebo-controlled multicenter trial looked at 1,845 women, ages forty to sixty-five years old. Its focus was to evaluate the safety and efficacy of oral estradiol with progesterone for the treatment of postmenopausal women with vasomotor symptoms, as well as to evaluate the hormone therapy's effect on the endometrium, or lining, of the uterus.

- Trial participants were randomized to receive varying doses of daily oral estradiol with progesterone or a placebo.

- Some study participants experienced vascular adverse effects, including coronary heart disease and deep vein thrombosis.

- After one year, there was no excess growth of the uterine lining or endometrial hyperplasia, *and* the women with hot flashes experienced meaningful improvements in their symptoms.

- Based on these findings, Bijuva became the first FDA-approved oral bioidentical combination of estradiol with continuous progesterone formulation.

- The message was that this product, because the FDA deemed it "safe," was a better alternative to compounded hormone therapy products that women had been using after the WHI stoppage (more on compounded hormones following).

STUDY OF WOMEN'S HEALTH ACROSS THE NATION (SWAN)
Begun in 1994 and still continuing today, SWAN is an ongoing, multisite longitudinal, epidemiologic study designed to examine the health of women during their middle years.

- The study has shown that women with hot flashes had higher asymptomatic cardiovascular diseases, including greater aortic valve calcium deposits, arterial stiffness, and carotid artery thickness, than women who did not have hot flashes.

- The study also found that women who started hormone therapy treatment within the first ten years after menopause had increased protection against death and heart attacks, and no increased risk of stroke than those who did not use hormone therapy.

- SWAN, especially when combined with ELITE, shows that time is of the essence with regard to starting hormone therapy when it comes to protecting vascular and heart health.

Although study designs varied, the totality of the studies post-WHI show that hormone therapy is indeed health protective for postmenopausal women, particularly when started early after menopause. Specifically, hormone therapy has now been conclusively shown to benefit women's hearts, bones, sexual function, uterus, and breasts. Notwithstanding these great outcomes, more research using better hormone therapy regimens may be needed to better educate and convince medical professionals so that the lingering WHI conclusions can finally be put to rest.

COMPOUNDED BIOIDENTICAL HORMONES: SAFE AND EFFECTIVE

From a consumer standpoint, despite the antihormone panic, because of post-WHI studies as well as the positive clinical outcomes seen in their patients, a growing group of compounding pharmacists and "alternative" medicine doctors in the United States pushed back and started informing their menopausal patients about hormone therapy options that were different from the synthetic hormones used in the WHI and marketed by pharmaceutical companies. These practitioners were acutely aware of the

THE REGULATION OF COMPOUNDING PHARMACIES

Keep in mind: Although conventional doctors in the United States will often claim compounded medications are "dangerous" or "unregulated," in reality, all pharmacists and pharmacies engaged in compounding are subject to oversight by both federal and state authorities.

The **practice** of compounding is regulated by state boards of pharmacy, which set standards and regulations for the types of preparations compounded. In addition, the United States Pharmacopeial (USP) Convention and National Formulary issue standards that apply to compounding.

- The USP develops standards for the identity, quality, strength, and chemical purity of medicines, dietary supplements, and food ingredients that may be used in compounding preparations.

- The National Formulary provides oversight on quality assurance.

- Compliance with USP and National Formulary guidelines is considered the *minimum* standard of practice for compounders.

The **components used** in compounded formulations are then overseen by the United States Food and Drug Administration (FDA) and the United States Drug Enforcement Agency (DEA). The FDA has extensive oversight for the integrity and safety of the drugs (called active pharmaceutical ingredients) used in compounded preparations, while the DEA has oversight for any controlled substances used in the preparation of compounded medications. Compounding pharmacists are regulated by their state boards of pharmacy.

So, while the "final product" from a compounding pharmacy does not have an "FDA Approved" label on it, the products from compounding pharmacies are the result of extensive oversight by multiple state and federal regulatory bodies and are not even remotely "dangerous."

hundreds (some would say thousands) of years of safe use of natural hormone therapies we described in chapter 10. In addition, they correctly recognized the significant distinction between putting endocrine-disrupting man-made chemicals into a woman's body versus using hormones created from natural, nonanimal sources that, on a chemical and molecular level, are an identical match to that of the hormones our body used to make.

Referred to as "bioidentical," these hormones were introduced to the general public by Suzanne Somers in her 2004 book *The Sexy Years*. By 2005, information about them had reached millions of postmenopausal women who then started seeking these hormones from medical providers. Wyeth, which had lost billions of dollars in revenue after the WHI was stopped, decided to retaliate by submitting a citizen petition to the FDA asking for stronger regulation and federal supervision of compounding pharmacies producing these bioidentical hormone preparations, even though these pharmacies were already subject to oversight by their state boards as well as extensive federal regulations. Shortly thereafter, Somers published a second book, *Ageless*, which pushed the message on these bioidentical hormones even further. Wyeth was so incensed that it enlisted the help of the North American Menopause Society, which is sponsored by Wyeth, and together they complained to the American Medical Association (AMA). The AMA responded by passing a resolution in support of Wyeth and petitioned the US Congress, asking for more regulation of bioidenticals from the FDA.

Of note, when the acronym HRT is used, it may mean bioidentical hormones but it also often refers to synthetic hormones. BHRT always means only

bioidentical hormones. Both can be either commercial or compounded. Because the FDA does not approve compounded bioidentical hormones, most insurances do not cover these. Notwithstanding the pharmaceutical industry's attacks on compounded hormones or their lack of FDA approval, studies examining physiological data and clinical outcomes demonstrate that bioidentical hormones are associated with lower risks, including the risk of breast cancer and cardiovascular disease, and are more efficacious than their synthetic and animal-derived counterparts. For this reason, women should not fear bioidentical hormones provided by compounded pharmacies.

WHERE THINGS STAND TODAY

Despite the many positive reanalyses and new scientific studies of, as well as significant consumer demand for, hormone therapy, the WHI's continued legacy is an environment of circulating misinformation that has left women with a crisis of inertia due to science, politics, and corporate profit motives.

Physicians cannot get past the decades of high-profile studies that used synthetic hormones produced by Big Pharma and dosed in poor forms resulting in bad outcomes, and prestigious institutions such as Harvard, Stanford, and UCLA as well as leading cancer treatment centers continue to confuse, ignore, or falsely dismiss the differences between hormones that are foreign to the human body compared to hormones molecularly identical to our own hormones.

One of the biggest blocks to progress on the issue of hormone therapy stems from the fact that the medical-pharmaceutical complex's most significant profits come from treating the diseases of aging—not preventing them. So there remains incredible resistance to recognizing hormone therapy as an effective preventive for chronic disease. Add to this the incredible resistance to and continued misinformation on the use of compounded hormones, and we have barely moved beyond the post-WHI panic. We believe, however, this is starting to change.

Physicians and research organizations have shifted to offer weak support for using hormone therapy, but only FDA-approved options and to solely treat only "symptoms of menopause." This has come, in part, due to pressure from the Endocrine Society, a professional, international medical organization founded in 1916. They have stated:

> The widespread availability of FDA-approved bioidentical hormones produced in monitored facilities demonstrates a high quality of safety and efficacy in trials; therefore, there is no rationale for the routine prescribing of unregulated, untested, and potentially harmful custom-compounded bioidentical hormone therapies. Clinicians are encouraged to prescribe FDA-approved hormone products according to labeling indications and to avoid custom-compounded hormones.

In 2022, the North American Menopause Society released a position statement declaring that hormone therapy remains the most effective treatment for hot flashes and genitourinary syndromes of menopause and can prevent bone loss and fracture. They also stated that these benefits outweigh the risks for most healthy symptomatic women who are aged younger than sixty years and within ten years of menopause onset, but when used for the management of persistent hot flashes or worsening osteoporosis, hormone therapy can be continued beyond age sixty-five.

Despite these tepid statements giving limited support for hormone therapy, there is more encouraging evidence that a bigger shift may be afoot.

The American Heart Association's current position statement on hormone therapy states:

> [C]urrent recommendations from leading specialty societies endorse the use of [hormone therapy] in recently menopausal women with appropriate indications. The evidence supports cardiovascular benefit for [hormone therapy] initiated early among women with premature or surgical menopause and within ten years of menopause in women with natural menopause. *The benefits of [hormone therapy] (i.e, including lower rates of diabetes, reduced insulin resistance, and protection from bone loss) appear to outweigh risks for the majority of early menopausal women* [emphasis added]. Perimenopausal women should be provided individualized guidance on [hormone therapy] and options for treatment, particularly when [hot flashes] are present.

THE MISSING PIECE TO HEALTHY AGING

If hormone therapy were harmful to the health of postmenopausal women, its massive reduction in use should have resulted in an improvement in women's health, but as we laid out in chapter 1, women are *not* aging well. On top of painful and life-disrupting symptoms and poor metabolic health, during and after the menopausal transition women continue to be at the greatest risk for osteoporosis and bone fractures, certain cardiovascular events, cognitive decline and disease, certain cancers, auto-immune diseases, and various mental health conditions. What's worse is that, for every decade after age fifty, these changes accumulate and amplify the degenerative processes such that women decline in dramatic fashion compared to men.

There is no dispute over how women's sex hormones exert crucial influence on and control over the hundreds of physiologic signals upon which their whole body health and disease risk depend. In addition, nearly every study on hormone therapy, including those with a negative bias or that express concerns and promote limitations on its use, demonstrates that its usage has a positive effect on mortality. Notwithstanding all of this, currently there are no trials with endpoints seeking to identify hormone therapy as preventive therapy to restore and maintain women's health, let alone head-to-head safety trials comparing compounded bioidentical hormones to FDA-approved—let alone synthetic—hormones. Women deserve better.

Aging with a completely different trajectory *is* possible: With hormones extended or restored systemically and in the correct physiologic ranges, women have an incredible chance to retain a healthy brain, nervous system, muscles, ligaments, joints, tendons, bones, sleep quality, mood, memory, cognition, sexual function, libido, and more. Although lifestyle factors such as midlife nutrition, digestion, sufficient sleep, stress management, appropriate movement, and self-care are critical to helping reduce the symptoms and side effects of hormone loss due to menopause, the *only* thing that can replicate the work of our hormones is . . . the hormones themselves. While the medical guidelines have barely changed, that does not mean that hormone therapy is not a safe and effective intervention to preserve women's health.

You deserve to thrive as you age, and we want to help you make that happen. Knowing what would be best for you requires knowing what your options are, how to find a skilled and knowledgeable health care provider, and what options you have if your personal circumstances require you to consider nonhormonal options.

CHAPTER TWELVE

MENOPAUSE CARE A TO Z

TO HELP YOU ADVOCATE FOR YOURSELF better and protect your health, we are going to take the next two chapters to cut through all the noise and offer you a complete look at all therapies typically offered to midlife women, including those for whom hormone therapy is an option (this chapter) and those who truly fall into one of the categories contraindicated for hormones and who may need alternative options (chapter 13). Regardless of where you think you fall on the hormone therapy spectrum, we urge all women to read both this and the following chapter to become as fully informed on the subject as possible.

As we stated in chapter 10, the concept of hormone therapy for menopausal women is often presented and discussed as if there were a single, standardized, uniform option, sort of like buying ibuprofen, whether branded or generic, in 200 mg tablets and just taking the dose you need. Unfortunately, that is not the case with hormone therapy, as it comes in many forms and regimens, which makes the topic confusing for many. And, for some women, hormone therapy is not an option and so nonhormonal options are needed that can, at a minimum, mitigate the symptoms that arise from states of hormone deprivation.

To add to the confusion, some doctors offer women—in and after the menopausal transition—treatment options that contain no hormones but present these options as if they will address the root issues that are a consequence of hormone loss. Add that what you are offered is usually dependent on your *provider's* treatment goals, which may be different from *your* health goals. And this doesn't consider how some doctors still perceive hormone therapy as dangerous or, even worse, do not even know what hormones do for our health beyond fertility. Consequently, it can be near impossible to receive the most effective treatment for your whole body health and disease prevention.

To provide you with the most comprehensive guide, we start with an overview of all therapies commonly offered to women, both nonhormonal and hormonal (and for purposes of brevity, we refer to hormone therapy going forward as "HRT").

NONHORMONAL THERAPIES

Although HRT is the most effective treatment for health issues presented by hormone deprivation, there are many physicians who will refuse to prescribe it simply because of a lack of training and/or misinformation and misunderstanding, or because they are unwilling to make a long-term investment in you to manage your HRT journey. When *non*hormonal therapies are offered by medical providers, they fall into one of two categories: nonpharmacological and pharmacological, both with a treatment goal of symptom management only. And while nonhormonal treatments can reduce discomfort and may improve a woman's quality of life, they will not signal the internal genomic actions previously controlled by sex hormones.

Science-Backed Nonhormonal and Nonpharmacological Treatments

- Acupuncture
- Cognitive behavioral therapy (CBT)
- Dressing in layers, using cooling pads

- Exercise
- Herbs and supplements
- Hypnosis
- Mindfulness, breathing, restorative exercise
- Nerve blocks: Injections of anesthetic into the sympathetic nerve fibers of the neck to disrupt neural temperature regulation can reduce hot flashes
- Plant-based nutrition: Eating heavy amounts of soy and other "phyto-estrogen" foods can occupy the estrogen receptor and downregulate deficiency symptoms
- Weight loss

Oftentimes, whether HRT is contraindicated or not, many doctors will first offer women nonhormonal pharmacological-based treatments. Again, as with the options listed previously, these are for symptom management and will not restore the functions controlled by hormones.

Nonhormonal Pharmacological Treatments

- Anticonvulsants, such as gabapentin, Klonopin, and pregabalin
- Antidepressants/antianxiety medications
- Antihistamines and OTC pain medications
- Antihypertensives, such as clonidine
- Asthma inhalers and oral asthma drugs
- Benzodiazepine sedative hypnotics, such as Ativan, ProSom, Restoril, Valium, and Xanax
- Bisphosphonates, such as Actonel, Boniva, Fosamax, and Reclast
- Nerve pain medications, such as nortriptyline
- NK3R antagonists, such as fezolinetant/Veozah and new options on the horizon
- Non-benzodiazepine hypnotics, such as Ambien, Lunesta, and Sonata
- SSRIs (selective serotonin reuptake inhibitors), such as Lexapro, Prozac, and Zoloft
- SNRIs (serotonin and norepinephrine reuptake inhibitors), such as Cymbalta and Effexor
- Statins

It is important to note that pharmacological drugs rarely come without unintended consequences. For this reason, it is imperative to investigate side effects and make an informed decision about these interventions if any are offered to you. For example, benzodiazepine drugs can be habit-forming and cause suicidal ideation; statins can increase the risk of diabetes and cause muscle atrophy and brain fog; and NK3R antagonists can cause elevated liver enzymes and put women at risk for nonalcoholic metabolic fatty liver disease. In most instances, you have better options than those that put your health at risk.

A third class of drugs that enters into treating hormone loss are selective estrogen receptor modulators, or SERMs. These are oral nonsteroidal medications that act as an estrogen agonist or antagonist depending on the target tissue of the body. As an agonist, SERMs bind to estrogen receptors, producing a similar response to that of estradiol. As an antagonist, SERMs bind to the receptors and altogether stop the receptors from producing a response. SERMs are most commonly used with estrogen-positive breast cancer but different SERMs have different patterns of action in various areas of the body. Common SERMs are conjugated estrogens with bazedoxifene (Duavee), ospemifene (Osphena), raloxifene (Evista), tamoxifen (Soltamox), and toremifene (Fareston). These may be offered to women concurrently with HRT but they will reduce the hormones' efficacy.

HORMONE-BASED THERAPIES

What constitutes hormone therapy or gets called HRT by medical providers varies significantly depending on someone's background. To some doctors, a birth control pill or even an IUD given to a fifty-year-old woman is HRT. To others, giving a woman only high doses of testosterone is a proper approach to HRT. For others yet, it may be a pill, a patch, or both! The reality is that the biochemistry, metabolism, and physiologic effects of the various therapies considered to be HRT also vary widely and, accordingly, have meaningfully different risks and benefits. For this reason, to give you the best understanding of the A to Z of hormone therapy and what might be right for you, we start with a review of terms and characteristics that are relevant to evaluating any particular option. At the end of this section, you'll find some easy rules to help make sense of it all.

Hormone Therapy Nuances to Know

While some proponents may argue that any and all hormone products are good for hormone therapy, when it comes to hormone restoration, that is simply not the case. It is really no different than understanding how not all calories are the same—such as how 300 calories from a donut are wildly different nutritionally than 300 calories from a chicken breast. For this reason, we want to give you a deep look at the different forms of hormone therapy, specifically by examining molecular type and sourcing, manufacturing, regulatory approval, area of action, hormone type, and more.

MOLECULAR TYPE

The active molecules in hormone therapy are either *synthetic* or *bioidentical* (also called body-identical or biomimetic). Despite the use of the term *natural* for either type, both synthetic and bioidentical hormones are modified or manufactured in a lab. Synthetic hormones are "hormone-like" molecules produced (or synthesized) in a laboratory from a "natural" source but that have a slightly altered chemical structure from the actual hormone found in the body. Bioidentical hormones are hormone molecules that are also made from a natural source but that are structurally (chemically) identical to the "natural" hormones they are intended to replace.

The molecular type matters because bioidentical hormones replicate the exact chemical structure of naturally produced human hormones (estrogen, progesterone, testosterone, etc.), and so they "plug into" the hormone receptor to create a proper signal just like a body-produced hormone does. A bioidentical hormone's communication is like having a conversation with another human. With synthetic hormones, it is like trying to carry on a conversation with Siri from your phone; some things are going to be lost in translation even though it was created by humans.

MOLECULE SOURCING

Hormone therapies originate from either a plant, an animal source, or man-made chemical compounds, or combinations thereof. Plant-derived hormones result in bioidentical molecules when produced pharmacologically, whereas animal- and chemical-derived hormones have different chemical structures from human hormones. This means that although synthetic hormones can stimulate the receptor, the signal is altered and different from that which is delivered by bioidentical hormones. This can damage the receptor itself as well as lead to a cascade of abnormal and potentially dangerous outcomes, such as DNA damage and cancer.

MEDICAL MANUFACTURING

Some hormone therapies are "commercial" whereas others are "compounded." Commercial therapies are mass-produced, ready-made, and approved by the FDA, whereas compounded therapies are custom-made on an individual basis according to a prescription from a licensed health care provider. Although compounded products do not receive "FDA approval," the FDA regulates their base ingredients and components, and the labs and pharmacies processing them are subject to significant oversight by state pharmacy boards as well as the FDA and other federal agencies.

FDA "APPROVAL"

Many conventional physicians believe FDA approval makes a hormone therapy "safe" compared to a compounded one. This, however, is a misguided perception. The purpose of FDA approval for a drug is to prove that a specific substance can treat a condition. Most of the time, FDA-approved drugs are man-made, not natural, and so an approval process ensures that they are not only safe but also effective for that specific indication. For example, FDA approval is needed for the route of administration of IV salt in water (a.k.a. saline) for dehydration because it is the route of administration and dose/volume in that IV that has to be proven to be safe and effective.

Compounded drugs are bioidentical natural substances and their safety is already known—FDA approval is not needed to prove it.

To require FDA approval for something natural and inherently safe would be like saying administering water for dehydration would need FDA approval. Compounding provides greater dosage and ingredient flexibility to meet the needs of the individual user. For example, the FDA-approved Prometrium is a form of bioidentical progesterone suspended in peanut oil and the capsules contain D&C Yellow No. 10, FD&C Red No. 40, and FD&C Yellow No. 6. It also only comes in 100 mg or 200 mg doses per

capsule. Some women are allergic to one or more of these ingredients and/or need a different dosage. As a result, they are unable to be prescribed the FDA-approved Prometrium and require and benefit from a compounded form of progesterone.

AREA OF ACTION

Hormone therapies can be applied and act either "locally" or "systemically." Locally delivered hormones are usually applied vaginally and signal only the hormone receptors in that area.

Because its actions are limited, local hormone therapy is an important and viable option for genitourinary problems such as vaginal dryness, painful intercourse, incontinence, and recurrent urinary tract infections when systemic hormone therapy is contraindicated (for example, for cancer patients).

Systemic hormones, on the other hand, initiate the hormone signals at all receptors throughout the body and stimulate the global genomic processes needed for optimal health and disease protection.

PRODUCT AVAILABILITY

Despite the incredible power of hormone therapy, surprisingly, some versions are available as over-the-counter options, either as DIY consumer supplements or as low-dose "professional" products. It should be obvious that something available without a prescription does not have the same efficacy and safety that prescription hormones do. In fact, hormone therapy should never be a DIY or consumer-driven option without regular oversight by a licensed medical provider deeply trained in hormone therapy.

VARIOUS WAYS SYSTEMIC HORMONE THERAPY IS DOSED

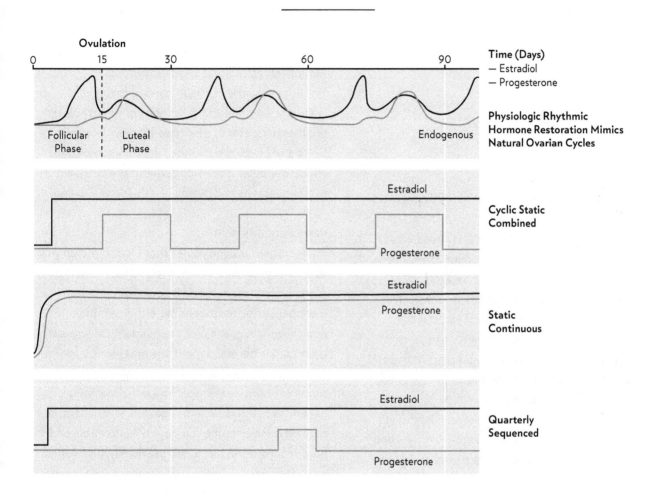

ESTROGEN TYPE

As described in chapter 2, there are three main types of estrogen: estrone, estradiol, and estriol. In terms of hormone therapy, estrone in any form is a concern because it results in thrombotic events (clotting) and because it primarily stimulates estrogen receptor alpha (ER-α), which results in uncontrolled proliferation or growth of tissues.

Likewise, use of estriol in hormone therapy, most often found in formulations called Bi-Est, or more rarely Tri-Est, is also a concern. Estriol is the most dominant estrogen in pregnancy and one of its roles is to deliberately downregulate the immune system to prevent rejection of the DNA from the sperm as part of the fetus. When a menopausal woman uses systemic estriol, the result is replication of this low immune environment of pregnancy. In addition, estriol primarily stimulates ER-β (estrogen receptor beta), which results in putting a brake on the actions of estradiol, thereby diluting its benefits. Finally, the

NOTE ON ESTRIOL

Many physicians primarily use systemic estriol because they believe it is "safer" than estradiol, namely that it is cancer protective (and estradiol is not). This misguided belief is based on a single study from 1966 that examined the urine of women with and without cancer and compared that to the urine of pregnant women. The researchers concluded that since estriol is the highest estrogen during pregnancy and pregnant women do not get breast cancer (not true, actually!) and that six of the cancer patients had low urine estriol levels, estriol must be protective against breast cancer. From this (weak) data, much research has adopted this presumption and run with it. As we now know from more recent and better studies, estradiol can be cancer protective as well. Even more important, it is unnecessary to give a woman systemic estriol because if she has enough systemic estradiol she will make whatever estriol is "needed" by the body. Given estriol's unbalanced estrogen receptor stimulation as well as its downregulation of the immune system, using it as systemic hormone therapy is not helpful to postmenopausal women's health.

systemic use of estriol raises the risk of what's referred to as "receptor competition" where estriol edges out estradiol. Overall, the use of systemic estriol is unnecessary as a supplementary estrogen because the body will convert estradiol to estriol, if needed.

Ultimately, the estrogen needed for aging our best is 17-beta estradiol. Estradiol does not create clotting or other risks, acts in a balanced fashion between ER-α and ER-β, and provides the only stimulus for critical genomic actions throughout the body, ensuring homeostasis and overall health and well-being.

PROGESTOGEN TYPE

Progestogens are molecules that bind to the progesterone receptor and attempt to initiate the actions of the progesterone made by our ovaries before menopause. Progestogens are either synthetic and called "progestins" or are bioidentical and just called progesterone. Progestins are typically found in birth control pills but are also present in some forms of hormone therapy. The most common generic progestins are etonogestrel, levonorgestrel, medroxyprogesterone (Depo, MPA, Provera), and norethindrone. As discussed previously, progestins are not a molecular match to a woman's own progesterone and so react with the progesterone receptor in a way that is disruptive to the endocrine system, creating altered signals shown to contribute to breast cancer, among other conditions.

Conversely, bioidentical progesterone is produced from a plant source and is chemically and structurally identical to human progesterone, so it acts appropriately at the receptor and is actually protective at the breast and other areas in the body.

CONSTRUCTION: SINGLE OR MIXED

Hormone therapies can be constructed as isolated hormones, paired or mixed "cocktails," or blends. Progestogen-only therapy is the most common for perimenopausal women as it is easy to obtain and often sold over the counter in the United States. Symptom relief may happen initially but the therapy will eventually stop working because progesterone receptors decline without adequate estradiol. When dosed too high, progestogen-only therapy can increase anxiety and cause water retention and weight gain, but when dosed correctly, bioidentical progesterone can improve mood and sleep.

Testosterone-only therapies for women require a very careful approach because, unfortunately, they can result in supraphysiologic, or unnaturally high, levels of testosterone in the body. The risks from this include impaired liver function, cardiovascular changes, impaired bone remodeling, breast cancer, endometrial cancer, and behavioral and personality changes. In addition, the testosterone receptor shares a cell wall with the estradiol receptor, which means it can block part of estradiol's actions. For this reason, testosterone therapy should not be initiated until after estradiol has been optimized. When dosed and timed correctly, however, testosterone can improve a woman's mood, motivation, and sexual function as well as bone, brain, and breast health.

Estrogen-only regimens are rare but surprisingly still used in very conventional medical circles. If a woman still has her uterus, the risk of an estrogen-only therapy is uncontrolled proliferation, or growth, of endometrial tissues. If a woman does not have her uterus and is given only estrogen, she does not receive the important stimulation of the p53

PREGNENOLONE: THE MOTHER HORMONE IS NOT A VALID HORMONE THERAPY FOR MENOPAUSE

A strange trend among some doctors is prescribing pregnenolone rather than prescribing sex hormones for postmenopausal women. Pregnenolone is a steroid hormone synthesized from cholesterol and is naturally produced in the body by the mitochondria of adrenal glands and ovaries. While pregnenolone is considered the "mother hormone" from which our sex and other steroid hormones are made, giving it as hormone therapy is not an effective approach because there is no way to insert it into the mitochondria of the adrenal glands and ovaries. There is no research showing supplemental pregnenolone will address the loss of genomic signaling due to menopausal hormone deficiency and, thus, it is not a valid substitution for HRT.

---

cancer tumor suppressor signal, nor does she receive the important protective actions of progesterone on the brain, skeletal and smooth muscles, immune response, inflammation, and tissue regeneration.

In addition to giving each hormone on its own, an increasingly common practice is to deliver hormones as a mixed "cocktail" in a single formulation. Whether estrogen paired with testosterone, estrogen paired with progesterone, or even all three together, the use of mixed hormone "cocktails" in one formula presents its own set of problems. As noted previously, when testosterone is prematurely coupled with estrogen, part of the estrogen receptor gets occupied by testosterone, thereby blocking up to one-third of the estrogen from reaching its receptor. This often makes achieving desired estradiol levels difficult. In addition, mixing hormones in one cocktail formulation makes it impossible to identify which, if any, hormone may need adjustment, and this will prevent women from optimizing their hormone therapy for the best outcome.

DOSE FREQUENCY

Depending on the pharmacokinetics of a hormone therapy—meaning the amount of time taken for its absorption, bioavailability, distribution, metabolism, and excretion—the frequency with which hormone therapy can be taken ranges from once daily to once weekly to even multiple times in a day or week. Sadly, many hormone therapy providers do not take pharmacokinetics into account and will prescribe an estrogen with a half-life of twelve hours once a day, with the result being that women will be estrogen replete for only half the day and deprived of estrogen for the other half. The best person to discuss the pharmacokinetics of your hormone therapy with is your pharmacist.

DOSING REGIMEN

Hormone therapy can be dosed with different regimens depending on the types of hormones being used. For example, a woman might take the exact same dose every day, which is referred to as *static dosing*. Alternatively, a hormone therapy dose may change daily throughout the cycle, called *rhythmic dosing*. If you go back to the changes in hormone production across the menstrual cycle (see images on pages 34 and 35), you will realize that static dosing does not align with how a woman's body made hormones before menopause and therefore provides an unnatural pattern of hormones in the body. Static dosing also does not allow optimal progesterone receptors to be produced, which results in inadequate cell apoptosis and a higher chance of breast cancer initiation and recurrence. In addition, static dosing can prompt receptors to downregulate due to constant exposure without changing volume. Healthy women in their twenties and thirties have monthly hormone rhythms that play critical roles in directing the important genomic sequences for whole body health. Accordingly, rhythmic dosing is the only form of HRT that attempts to approximate nature by following the rhythmic timing of hormones in the body as they had been produced before menopause and maintain those genomic actions for whole body health.

DOSING COMBINATION

In the vast majority of instances, progesterone and estrogen are (and should be) taken together. As discussed in chapters 2 and 3, both of these hormones are essential for a woman's whole body health, whether the uterus is intact or not. Even more important, they have a synergistic relationship with the ebb and flow, which is physiologically relevant to the genomic sequences needed for healthy aging. To this end, before the menopausal transition, progesterone is present cyclically only during the luteal phase, or the second two weeks of a woman's monthly cycle.

While estrogen should be taken every day of the month, there are two methods to dosing

THE GREAT PROGESTERONE DEBATE:
TO CYCLE OR NOT

As we stated earlier, cycling progesterone mimics the way a woman's body produced progesterone before menopause. This is key because continuous progesterone exposure presents a variety of negative consequences that threaten a woman's ability to age healthfully. That said, cycling progesterone will initiate a monthly bleed and if there's one thing that women (mistakenly) celebrate in menopause, it is the cessation of menstruation. We believe that can change once women realize that the uterus and its monthly bleed is a barometer indicating how the rest of the body is functioning. A scheduled, normal bleed tells us whether we are in an optimum state of health. To use hormone therapy with a uterus and not have a period shows a lack of optimal function. Although most conventional doctors will resist reinitiating a uterine cyclic bleed in menopause, it is truly up to the patient to decide. Rather than seeing it as an inconvenience, when women understand what a regular cycle represents, they tend to embrace the idea, though some may still have questions, the most common being:

- **Will the bleed be comparable to what I had before menopause?** Not necessarily. A cyclic hormone therapy bleed is not a replication of whatever you had premenopause; rather, it is managed and scheduled so it lasts three to five days, has mild to moderate flow, and comes with no PMS or cramping. If it falls outside these parameters, then your provider will manipulate the HRT dose and regimen to craft the bleed into an optimal presentation.

- **Does a monthly bleed with hormone therapy restore fertility?** Not for a menopausal woman who has lost her ovarian egg reserve; however, cycling progesterone can restore fertility for premenopausal women struggling with hormone sufficiency.

- **Will a monthly bleed cause anemia?** Not by its practice as designed; however, if the bleeding is excessive and uncontrolled, as could be the case with an unhealthy or unstable uterus or when estrogen levels need adjustment, it could lead to anemia (and this is no different than the premenopausal risk). Exceptions could be women who have dangerously low ferritin before initiating hormone therapy, in which case, any bleeding could cause anemia.

- **Are there cases in which cyclic hormones should not be used?** In very rare instances, some women may have severe premenstrual dysphoric disorder (PMDD) with hormone fluctuations. Even in these cases, these symptoms are often due to hormones being too low, so best practice is to start with physiologic rhythmic hormone therapy and adjust dosing to manage symptoms.

- **What happens if cycling hormones does not produce a bleed?** This can happen when women start HRT very late and long after menopause when receptors are very flat and not functioning; it is not problematic as long as the uterine lining is monitored. With younger menopausal women who do not bleed, a dosing adjustment to taper the progesterone dose more abruptly is usually all that is needed. Still, it is not dangerous, but rather a sign that the hormone therapy simply needs to be modified. This exemplifies why having a period and utilizing vaginal ultrasounds as needed are the best monitors of women's health.

progesterone alongside estrogen: continuously, meaning it is taken every day of the month, or cyclically, meaning it is taken only for the same two weeks every monthly cycle. (Note that some hormone therapy providers choose an entirely random schedule for progesterone, such as five days on, two days off, or three months on, one month off. There is no physiologic or medical basis for this and any such dosing recommendations should be a red flag that the provider is not providing evidence-based care.)

Dosing progesterone in a cyclic regimen designed to mimic the normal luteal phase before menopause is the preferred standard of care according to UpToDate, the most trusted evidence-based clinical decision support resource used by medical providers. Notwithstanding this, the most common hormone therapy dosing combination is to give women a progestogen continuously at the same dose every day right alongside estrogen. This does not come without costs. Aside from diverting away from our natural physiology, continuous progestogen hormone therapy use has been linked to an increased risk of cardiovascular events, less protection for brain health, increased risk for dementia and mild cognitive impairment, increased risk of destabilizing the uterus and causing breakthrough bleeding, and increased cancer risk. In addition, continuously blunting estradiol with progestogen over time ends up downregulating the estrogen receptor due to never having a robust level of estradiol on its own.

You might be wondering why a provider would ignore physiology let alone the published standard of care and expose women to the potential risks of continuous progesterone. It all comes down to the fact that, if a woman has a uterus, cycling progesterone will result in a withdrawl bleed. Yes, you read that right. Hormone therapy that cycles progesterone will create a regular, monthly uterine bleed. Because women tend to celebrate the loss of their menstrual cycle, most do not want any uterine bleed to return. Likewise, doctors have been taught that bleeding after menopause is dangerous and they do not want to have to manage a woman's health to this extent. To this we say, it is time to reframe how we view the uterine cycle. For women of any age, it is a vital sign that should be embraced as an indicator of whole body health. Remember, it is the up-and-down rhythm of our sex hormones and the uterine cycle that results that offer the strongest protections from cancer because it is the only way to activate the p53 tumor-suppressor gene.

DELIVERY METHOD

Delivery of hormone therapy varies significantly. Each hormone may be given transdermally (through the skin) using creams, gels, oils, sprays, and patches; as an injection (intramuscular or subcutaneous); orally (pills, lozenges, and drops); as a suppository (inserted into the rectum, vagina, or urethra); as an intrauterine device; or as pellets (solid, rice-shaped compounds inserted under the skin). Some hormones are better delivered in one form versus others and each delivery method has its pros and cons, depending on the hormone being given. For example, studies show that, when taken orally, estradiol increases inflammatory markers and clotting factors in the body, putting women at higher risk of dangerous blood clots and stroke, among other things. Estradiol taken through the skin, however, does not present these same risks.

An Evolving Landscape

Okay, whew! This was a significant amount of complex information, but we really want you to feel fully informed and able to gain fluency in the world of therapies available for women in and past the menopausal transition. Because the options available to women continue to change and because many of these options have important nuances that need to be considered, we have included a table at the end of this chapter for you to reference as you work to find the best therapy for you and your goals. Additionally, we will provide updates to this data via a reference web page.

HORMONE THERAPY: BASIC GUIDELINES

Although we are reluctant to distill hormone therapy down to a single list of best practices, we do want to provide you with some basic rules and guidance. At a very minimum, follow these points for hormone therapy:

Do

- Use **only bioidentical forms** of estradiol and progesterone
- Use both estradiol and progesterone, but not in the same formulation
- Cycle your progesterone, two weeks off and two weeks on
- Choose hormone therapy able to achieve pre-menopausal physiologic levels
- Choose rhythmic dosing of your hormones

Do Not

- Use oral estrogens
- Use estriol
- Use pellets of any kind
- Use cocktails or mixed delivery
- Have poor compliance, such as skipping or changing doses from what is prescribed

SUPPLEMENTS TO AVOID WHEN USING HORMONE THERAPY

Unbeknownst to many women, common herbal supplements often contain ingredients that can compete and interact negatively with hormone therapy. Anything marketed toward midlife women usually includes one or more of these ingredients because they can act as phytoestrogens or progesterone. Because using these will make optimizing your hormone therapy difficult, it is recommended that you avoid the following when using hormone therapy:

- Anise
- Black cohosh
- Curcumin/turmeric above 500 mg
- Diindolylmethane/indole-3-carbinol (DIM/I3C)
- Evening primrose oil
- Flax in large amounts
- Ginkgo
- Maca
- Schisandra
- *Selaura* nutritional supplement
- Selective estrogen receptor modulators (SERMs)

- Soy products
- St. John's wort
- Tribulus
- Vitex
- Wild yam

Other supplements and herbals marketed toward midlife women that *can help* address uncomfortable symptoms and that are not hormone-mimicking are fine, and they include:

- Lemon balm
- Melatonin
- Omega-3s
- Passionflower
- Pycnogenol
- Retinol
- Valerian
- Vitamin E

HORMONE THERAPY IS NOT A SET-IT-AND-FORGET-IT PROPOSITION

No matter how confident you feel in your choice of provider and hormone therapy regimen, one thing we cannot stress strongly enough is that no hormone therapy should be seen as a "set-it-and-forget-it" pursuit. As we age, our bodies change, our weight and metabolic health may change (for better or for worse), we go through seasons of new stress (sometimes acute, sometimes chronic), we have illnesses or surgeries, and more. Each change can alter our body's needs as well as its ability to absorb, metabolize, and respond to hormones. Think back to your younger years and how shifts in your health might have shifted your menstrual cycle or altered your PMS. Using therapies to extend the presence of hormones in our bodies as we age is no less susceptible to the shifts that occurred with our naturally made hormones before menopause. For this reason, know that over the years, it is not a failure of hormone therapy if you need to adjust or change your dosing, method, or other aspects of your regimen. In fact, it is normal and common. By using the knowledge you are gaining coupled with the partnership and oversight of a skilled provider, you will be able to navigate this changing landscape just fine. That said, we are proponents of not guessing but rather testing to see how your hormone therapy is being handled by your body. To that end, we provide a list of tests we recommend and utilize regularly (see appendix C, page 178).

BEING A HEALTHY HOST FOR HORMONE THERAPY

Hormone therapy is just as powerful as the hormones our body used to produce in robust amounts and, for that reason, it is important that, when using hormone therapy, we give it an optimal working environment— a healthy body.

Ideally, a woman who chooses hormone therapy:

- Is not currently using any birth control or IUD
- Maintains a healthy, non-obese weight
- Has strong metabolic health
- Has good gut health
- Has a stable uterus (if present)

Realistically, given the burdens of time, hormone loss, and general aging, many women come into this life stage struggling in one or more of these areas. Does that mean hormone therapy is not an option? No, definitely not. What it does mean, however, is that whether before or concurrently with starting hormone therapy, you need to give attention to these issues.

Evaluating your lifestyle and metabolic health are important for all midlife women. Removing endocrine-disrupting chemicals is key. These are man-made toxins or products that resemble many of our hormones and trick the body, bind to receptors, and don't let go from the receptor site like a natural hormone would, thereby eliciting a cascade of aberrant abnormalities. Chemicals such as per- and polyfluoroalkyl substances (PFAs), bisphenol A (BPA), polychlorinated biphenyl (PCB), phthalates, pesticides, and herbicides are the most common in our environment and important to eliminate. Having the right amount of fiber to keep your gut microbiome diverse, robust, and working daily is also key. Eliminate alcohol and the use of any OTC medications that burden the liver. Essentially, just living a low-inflammation lifestyle by eating optimal protein, healthy fats, and intentional carbohydrates; staying active; managing stress; and prioritizing sleep are the most beneficial investments you can make in your hormone therapy experience.

If you are currently using birth control or an IUD, plan on withdrawing that before starting hormone therapy. Nutritionally, support your body with healthy fiber, such as resistant starch, and ensure you eat sufficient calories with animal protein and fats optimized. In addition, addressing common vitamin and mineral deficiencies that arise from the use of synthetic hormones is important. Start a good B-complex vitamin along with magnesium, zinc, and vitamin D and provide support for your liver via herbal teas or supplements such as milk thistle and dandelion root. If you suspect a heavy liver burden due to alcohol use or prescription medications, consider using a castor oil pack or sauna therapy.

In the appendices located at the back of this book, we have provided various supplemental information for you to use as you evaluate which hormone therapy, if any, aligns with your current health and long-term goals. In appendix B (page 175), we provide a detailed list of all market options offered as hormone therapy (current as of our publication date). In appendix C (page 178), we include information on the tests you need to track the performance of your hormone therapy, and in appendix D (page 180), we provide detailed tests that can be used to evaluate and track your metabolic health.

If you are still unsure about using hormone therapy, are waiting to initiate hormone therapy, or are concerned that you are not eligible for hormone therapy, the next chapter discusses contraindications, both absolute and relative, that exist for HRT and provides detailed information regarding alternative interventions available to women for healthy aging when hormone therapy is truly not an option or needs to be stopped.

HORMONE THERAPY DELIVERY METHODS: QUICK FACTS, BENEFITS, AND DRAWBACKS

	Quick Facts	Benefits	Drawbacks
Birth Control Pill	• Oral pill • Long-standing "standard of care" option • Conventional recommendation for women up to age 55	• Familiar intervention • Little resistance from physicians • Usually covered by insurance • Provides pregnancy protection	• Not actual hormones, acts as an endocrine disruptor • Significant risks to breast health and cancer • Makes measuring natural hormones, particularly FSH, in the blood difficult
IUD	Small T-shaped plastic device inserted into uterus	• Set it and forget it • Lasts 3 to 10 years • Provides pregnancy protection	• Not real hormones (synthetics or nonhormonal), thus no protection from hormone deficiency • Effects are systemic despite providers' claims

	Quick Facts	Benefits	Drawbacks
IUD (continued)			• Breakthrough bleeding/spotting is common; can make periods heavier • Copper acts as a foreign estrogen, altering gene expression and displacing natural estrogens from estrogen receptors, thereby negatively affecting breast tissue and disrupting ovulation • Can fall out or puncture uterus
Vaginal Hormones	• Offered as cream, capsule, or suppository • Usually estradiol, estriol, or DHEA	• Fast acting; quick comfort • May provide urinary symptom benefits, including prevention of recurrent UTIs, overactive bladder, and urge incontinence • Can use when systemic HRT is contraindicated, but nonhormonal approaches are still first-line choice for managing vaginal issues during/after breast cancer treatment; among women with estrogen-dependent breast cancer history experiencing urogenital symptoms, vaginal estrogen reserved for those unresponsive to nonhormonal remedies • Low risk of transference	• Locally acting, thus nonsystemic and without whole body health benefits • Can be messy and difficult to use • Requires planning, thus inconvenient for spontaneity
Oral Estrogen, Progesterone Pill	• Easy to get • Usually covered by insurance	• Familiar form; easy to use • Can be customized via compounders • Oral progesterone can be an effective sleep aid	• Hormones are lost to digestive system, so higher dosing required • Less effective and difficult to optimize—impossible to predict what fraction makes it to the bloodstream • Oral estrogen is significantly associated with elevated inflammation

	Quick Facts	Benefits	Drawbacks
Oral Estrogen, Progesterone Pill (continued)			• Oral estrogen results in primarily estrone with high risk of deep vein thrombosis • Increases sex hormone–binding globulin, making less testosterone and estrogen available to act at receptors
Pellet	Rice-size implant put under the skin	• Simple, hands off • Longer duration: 3 to 4 months	• Physicians financially incentivized to push pellets • Surgical risks of bleeding, swelling, infection • No control of hormone levels; cannot adjust dose once implanted, even if side effects appear • Strong association with high triglycerides and liver problems • Offered by non-HRT providers (even dermatologists!) • Requires about 4 procedures annually • Sometimes provided as "combinations," making optimization difficult • Results in supraphysiologic levels of hormones, no sustained release • Extremely hard to determine blood levels to adjust amount of hormone in future doses • Known to negatively alter blood viscosity • May contain preservatives, degradation products, undesirable additives, or residual amounts of other drugs • May have substantial deviations from the prescribed dose

	Quick Facts	Benefits	Drawbacks
Troche/ Lozenge	Similar to a lozenge or cough drop; placed between cheek and gum to dissolve, releasing hormone slowly over time	• No transference concerns • Theoretically "bypasses" liver due to the high numbers of blood vessels in oral tissues and is thus directly absorbed and put immediately into circulation	• Not "liver sparing"; studies show more than 50% (up to 70%) of total troche dose is swallowed by the normal salivation process, which encounters stomach acids and first pass metabolism • Requires higher dosing as hormones are lost to digestion • Causes great fluctuations in hormone serum levels with spike, then low over 4 to 5 hours • Requires at least twice daily administration or 3 or 4 times for optimal results and to maintain adequate levels • Made from different bases, including polyethylene glycol, which can have a laxative effect and trigger severe allergic reactions such as anaphylaxis
Patch	Small adhesive with hormone on tiny pad in center	• Few side effects • Less conversion to estrone • Low clotting risk	• Low, nonphysiologic doses unable to fully protect whole body health • Standardized fixed dosing so cannot individualize to patient needs • Must change once or twice weekly and rotate on skin • Some react to the adhesives
Injection	• Intramuscular or subcutaneous • Given daily, weekly, or twice weekly	• Quick, effective replenishment of hormone levels • No hormone dosage is lost • Immediacy of delivery allows for quick adjustments to find optimal dose based on the body's response • Allows for greatest control of hormone levels	• Not all are comfortable with self-injections/needles • Injection schedule needs oversight to minimize variation in hormone levels (esters help with this)

	Quick Facts	Benefits	Drawbacks
Topical Cream/Gel	• Applied twice daily directly to the skin • Hormones are mixed in carrier base	• Absorbs slowly over time, delivering a steady dose • Can change carrier base for individual needs • Effective and simple • Provides steady continuous dose of hormones to avoid peaks and lows (which could cause mood swings and side effects)	• Compliance may wane due to volume of cream and drying time • Some base creams are better absorbed than others or contain ingredients some react to • Transference risk of passing the hormones on to other objects and people • Not all hormones reach the bloodstream (only 5% to 20%), which can reduce efficacy • Often made into combination treatment with multiple hormones, making dosing/treatment difficult

CHAPTER THIRTEEN

WHEN HORMONE THERAPY IS TRULY NOT AN OPTION

Managing Quality of Life in Midlife

WHILE HORMONE THERAPY IS THE MOST EFFECTIVE treatment for health issues presented by hormone deprivation, it can be truly medically contraindicated for some women. Most commonly, women with certain health conditions will be told to avoid HRT or proceed only under strict medical guidance. Depending on the condition, however, some may be only "relative contraindications," meaning that HRT may be possible, but a risk-benefit analysis is always warranted to individualize and optimize care.

UNDERSTANDING CONTRAINDICATIONS

In the world of health care, a contraindication is a condition that serves as a reason not to take a certain medical treatment. When it comes to HRT, there is a small list of conditions that some doctors will immediately declare as creating risk that makes a woman ineligible. In some of these instances, however, the evaluated risk must be balanced against whether nonhormonal therapies have been sufficient to treat the imperatives of hormone deficiency and whether HRT would significantly improve the patient's quality of life.

While there is a distinct set of conditions that may require HRT avoidance (see box at right), a "family history" of cancer is, hands down, the most common reason women self-exclude from pursuing HRT. Sadly, in the vast majority of instances, this is an overcorrection and flawed understanding of one's eligibility. For this reason, understanding and evaluating the difference between a *personal* cancer history and any *family* cancer history is required before making any decisions about HRT. In all instances, any history of cancer should always be approached with an individual-by-individual analysis weighing the risks of going without hormones versus the benefits of using hormone therapy.

Personal History of Cancer

If a woman has a personal history of cancer, what matters in the context of HRT is what type of cancer occurred. Metastatic estrogen receptor positive (ER+) breast, ovarian, endometrial, or uterine cancers are often considered disqualifiers from systemic HRT use. That said, locally applied topical hormone therapies, including lubricants using estradiol, DHEA, or testosterone, are often possible and can protect these women from the genitourinary issues that arise from hormone deprivation. Additionally, provided the cancer was not progesterone receptor positive (PR+), progesterone can be used to protect the body from further cancers for the vast majority of women and its use will be fine. If a woman is using a selective estrogen receptor modulator (SERM), such as Raloxifene or Tamoxifen, she can use systemic HRT but its efficacy will be reduced simply because these medications are competitive inhibitors of estrogen binding

MEDICAL CONDITIONS THAT MAY REQUIRE HRT AVOIDANCE

- Active acute chronic liver disease with dysfunction

- Active deep vein thrombosis (DVT), pulmonary embolism (PE), migratory thrombophlebitis (Trousseau's sign of malignancy), or factor V Leiden mutation *or* a history of these conditions, especially during pregnancy

- Active or recent (within the past year) arterial thromboembolic disease (such as transient ischemic attack, stroke, or myocardial infarction)

- Advanced coronary heart disease (atherosclerosis)

- Chronic active portal vein thrombosis

- Known or suspected metastatic estrogen receptor positive breast, ovarian, endometrial, or uterine cancer

- Pregnancy

- Severe and/or advanced cardiovascular, peripheral vascular, or cerebral vascular disease

- Severe hypertension

- Uncontrolled cardiac arrhythmias

- Undiagnosed vaginal bleeding after full investigation

to estrogen receptors. If a woman has been placed on an aromatase inhibitor such as Anastrozole, HRT is likely not an option.

Family History of Cancer

As stated earlier, too many women believe that any "family history" of cancer disqualifies them from HRT. This a flawed understanding of personal risk and HRT; it is very rarely, if ever, relevant. Any cancers of any family members where the onset was after the age of sixty are actually *not* equated to a "family history" of cancer relevant to HRT eligibility.

Cancer in *two or more* **first-degree** family members where onset was before age sixty does, however, constitute "family history" and may be relevant to HRT eligibility—but even in these instances more data are needed.

Provided a woman herself does not have preexisting cancer lesions, the benefits of HRT outweigh the risks—in most instances. Even more important, however, is the fact that among women with a family history, those who used HRT had a significantly lower risk for total mortality than did women who had never used HRT, including total cancer-related mortality.

At the end of the day, cancer is complex and highly dependent on toxin exposure and oxidative stress, so having a relative with it is not a determinant when it comes to HRT use, even if the relative's cancer was hormonal-driven or genetic testing shows you share high-risk genetic variations. If anything, using synthetic hormones or having low hormone levels such that you lack genomic signaling to stimulate the p53 tumor suppressor's actions are believed to be bigger risks for developing cancer. For this reason, in many instances, maintaining physiologic levels of hormones may actually be cancer protective.

Clotting Issues

Second to cancer, the next most common reason women believe they are ineligible for HRT use is due to having clotting disorders such as factor V Leiden, deep vein thrombosis, or pulmonary embolism. Similar to the considerations around cancer, nuance is needed here. Generally, the perceived risks around HRT and blood clots are often due to the route of administration (oral) and/or the form of HRT used (synthetic). By following best practices for HRT selection as outlined in chapter 12, the risk of clotting is minimal to nonexistent for the vast majority of women.

Factor V is a blood protein used in making clots. Factor V Leiden is a common variant that makes blood more likely to clot. If a woman has factor V Leiden or another clotting disorder but successfully brought a pregnancy to term, then her clotting risk is actually reduced with HRT due to estradiol and progesterone's effect of stabilizing fibrinogen and vascular tone and response. Specifically, transdermal estradiol is safe to use with most clotting disorders. Studies have shown that postmenopausal women with factor V Leiden have a three to four times greater risk of venous thromboembolism (VTE), a condition when a blood clot forms in a vein, than women their age who do not have factor V Leiden. When women with factor V Leiden took oral estrogen for HRT, their risk of VTE was magnified twenty-five times; however, women with factor V Leiden taking transdermal estrogen did not show any greater risk of clot than the expected three to four times higher risk level from their condition.

Relative Contraindications

A relative contraindication is a condition that makes a particular treatment or procedure possibly inadvisable but not absolutely so. For example, X-rays in pregnancy are relatively contraindicated (because of concern for the developing fetus) unless the X-rays are deemed wholly necessary. With respect to HRT eligibility, there are certain conditions that do require extra evaluation and a case-by-case analysis. Screening for challenges such as severely compromised metabolic health or conditions such as Lynch syndrome should be looked at alongside personal medical history, symptom severity, and lifestyle factors when making HRT eligibility determinations. In many instances, HRT can improve these conditions but special consideration and caution should be taken, nonetheless.

With respect to transdermal HRT creams, gels, and oils, one of the main relative contraindications is the potential for transference to family members and pets. Specifically, young, prepubescent children and/or small dogs (between 25 and 50 pounds [11.4 and 22.8 kg] in weight) in the home require extra precautions to prevent topical HRT from being "shared" inadvertently. In addition, for women who are more than 30 to 50 pounds (13.6 to 22.8 kg) overweight, transdermal HRT may have difficulty making its way to the hormone receptor, so a different form of HRT may be required.

Extremely poor gut health is another potential relative contraindication. Severe gut microbiome dysbiosis, significant permeability of the gut membrane (leaky gut), chronic IBS/IBD (whether diarrhea or constipation), chronic proton pump inhibitors (PPI) use or gastroesophageal reflux disease (GERD), and gastric bypass history all pose challenges to HRT

effectiveness. Accordingly, working on healing one's gut before or concurrent with starting HRT is essential.

Use of certain medications, such as antidepressant and antiseizure medications, can make HRT challenging but still possible. Often, the HRT provider will need to work with the particular medication prescriber to manage dosing adjustments that may be required given the positive influence of HRT on these conditions.

And although HRT has been shown to lower a woman's risk of various autoimmune conditions, systemic lupus erythematosus (SLE) is an outlier. HRT does have the potential to induce SLE flares. For this reason, women with active SLE disease or those with antiphospholipid (aPL) antibodies should not undertake HRT. HRT can, however, be used by women without active disease or antiphospholipid antibodies.

Finally, an unstable uterus usually requires some sort of imaging before beginning HRT. This means a pelvic or transvaginal ultrasound is recommended for women with the following:

- Abnormal ovarian cysts
- Adenomyosis
- History of unexplained dysfunctional uterine bleeding during the previous twelve months
- Polycystic ovary syndrome (PCOS) for more than thirty years
- Suspected or known history of fibroids
- Unexplained pelvic pain

None of these conditions is absolutely contraindicated for HRT but, in some instances, a hysterectomy may be advised by your doctor in order to gain the most benefit from HRT with no exacerbation of symptoms.

DOES AGE MATTER?

The prevailing narrative for much too long has been that if a woman is more than ten years past reaching menopause or over the age of sixty, she is not a candidate for HRT. In addition, women are told that once they reach the age of sixty, they should stop taking HRT. All of these beliefs could not be further from the truth and are based on poor data. In fact, no study has demonstrated a lack of safety with the use of non-oral bioidentical HRT in women over the age of sixty or more than ten years postmenopausal, and yet the standard (wrong) narrative is that HRT in these women is unsafe.

In the Women's Health Initiative study, although some of the subjects were older than sixty, not only were they metabolically unhealthy but also the HRT used was Premarin and Prempro, both synthetic hormones given orally that are now recognized as being potentially harmful to women, regardless of age. In the ELITE study, which is known as establishing a "timing hypothesis," bioidentical estradiol was used, but it was given orally. In this trial, the study endpoint was whether the walls of the carotid artery thickened, thereby increasing cardiovascular disease risk. When the results were split by age, the study showed that HRT started at or near the time of menopause provided significant reduction in cardiovascular disease but provided no such benefit when started more than ten years postmenopause.

Thankfully, despite the poor interpretation of these studies and the historical narrative cautioning women over the age of sixty from using HRT, both the North American Menopause Society and the American College of Obstetrics and Gynecology agree that the use of HRT should be individualized and *not* discontinued based solely upon age. In fact, because HRT is effective for osteoporosis and other hormone deprivation issues, such as genitourinary health, sleep, libido, skin and hair, mood and cognition, and more, these groups suggest that extended use of HRT is reasonable when the woman and her provider agree that the benefits outweigh any potential individual risks.

The truth is that women who spend an extended amount of time with depleted and insufficient hormones are already at greater risk for heart disease, cancer, clots, and more. For this reason, adjusting lifestyle to create a healthy host for HRT along with pre-initiation screening of cardiovascular status via tests such as a coronary artery calcium scan and a fractionated lipid panel that includes measuring lipoprotein(a) and fibrinogen are strongly recommended. If such test results are acceptable and metabolic health is not markedly poor, there is no reason for a woman of any age without any absolute contraindications to avoid HRT based simply on age or time since menopause.

CRUCIAL LIFESTYLE PURSUITS

Although symptom suppression without HRT may be a woman's initial concern, protecting against the long-term risks from hormone deprivation should be the real priority. To this end, nutrition and movement are the most tangible and influential "low-hanging" fruits in terms of accessible interventions, followed by addressing inflammation and stress to lower disease risk.

The everyday lifestyle pursuit for any woman—whether HRT eligible or not—should be combining an animal protein–centric diet with strength training and weight-bearing exercises to help optimize muscle mass and strength. Consuming enough healthy fats and healthy fiber to boost the gut microbiome are also important but have more individual variability. For some women, too much fiber can be constipating—and if there is one thing we want to keep moving as we age, it is our bowels! Play around with what works for you and do not worry about achieving any generally recommended guidelines around fiber.

After nutrition, one of the more impactful tools for metabolic and whole body health is movement. In particular, resistance or strength training should be part of every midlife woman's weekly routine. Muscle is critical for locomotion, bone health, immune function, and protecting against frailty, but muscle is also a "use it or lose it" tissue in the body. Exercising regularly has also been shown to remodel our lipids and improve heart health as well as act as a significant modulator of mood and sleep. If a sedentary lifestyle or joint deterioration causes pain for you, enlist the help of a physical therapist or other professional to build a progressive plan that can help you restore your exercise capacity. As we like to say to clients, "motion is lotion," and even if it is simply in little "exercise snacks" throughout the day (such as ten air squats at the top of every hour!), movement is an important key to healthspan.

The next most important lifestyle pursuit is addressing and minimizing inflammation. A low-toxin lifestyle that limits exposure to endocrine-disrupting chemicals, alcohol, smoking, and recreational drugs is essential. If past exposure is a concern, consider adding sauna and/or red light therapy to mitigate the oxidative stress caused by such exposure. Additionally, optimize your circadian rhythm and mitochondrial function with intentional habits around getting daily sunlight, keeping a regular sleep schedule, exercising regularly, managing stress, and prioritizing proper nutrient intake.

Finally, stress management is a crucial priority. We cannot eliminate stress, whether emotional, physical, social, or perceived, but we can help our body offload its effects. Interventions such as non-sleep deep rest protocols, meditation, prayer, gratitude journaling, and community engagement are all powerful methods to help our body switch out of a "fight-or-flight" state. If stress levels are so high that even these interventions are not sufficient, then consider supplemental support from adaptogens (more on these on page 160).

THERE'S NO MAGIC PILL, BUT SUPPLEMENTS CAN HELP

Although herbal supplements and adaptogens cannot fully make up for the loss of genomic signaling that hormones stimulated before menopause, they can be incredibly powerful interventions to help blunt, if not eliminate, the palpable symptoms as well as slow the risks from hormone loss in midlife. We provide options here, depending on the symptom that requires attention or the adaptogen being considered, but we do so with a few caveats:

1 **Beware of supplements labeled "proprietary blends,"** as there is no way of knowing the amounts of the individual ingredients in these supplements, making it impossible to identify which ingredient is helping or which ingredient may be causing a negative reaction.

2 **Be careful with herbs.** Herbs are *powerful* and should be used in the lowest doses. High dose use should include simultaneously monitoring kidney and liver markers in the blood.

3 **Do not use all of the options listed in each category following.** Choose one and try it for two to four weeks before moving on to something else. Supplements are best started one at a time so you can identify what may be improving, what may be worsening, and what may have no effect on your concerns.

4 **If you have an acute medical condition** or are regularly taking any prescription medications or over-the-counter drugs, be sure to check with your doctor or pharmacist about any potential interactions before starting any herbal supplements, adaptogens, or other nutraceutical.

Herbs for Common Symptoms

Herbal supplements, sometimes called botanicals, are a type of dietary supplement derived from plants, including their oils, roots, leaves, seeds, berries, or flowers. These products have been used for centuries with many different health benefits, some of which include reduction of or relief from the various uncomfortable symptoms that can affect women during and after the menopausal transition.

CATCHALL

- Selaura, a highly researched, twelve-ingredient blend that, when well sourced, is an natural alternative to HRT when it is contraindicated or refused.

HOT FLASH REDUCTION

- Black cohosh and vitamin E have been shown to be most effective for reducing menopausal hot flashes.

- Chasteberry (vitex) has been shown to reduce hot flashes.

- Fresh sage supplement has been shown to reduce hot flash intensity.

- Korean red ginseng, on its own, appears ineffective for hot flashes but *when combined with* black cohosh or red clover it may enhance their hot flash reduction effects.

- Pycnogenol (pine bark extract) has been shown to reduce hot flashes.

- Red clover appears effective at reducing hot flash frequency and intensity.

- Schisandra has been shown to support reductions in heart palpitations, sweating, and hot flash frequency.

INSOMNIA/FATIGUE

- The most commonly used herbs for insomnia as well as anxiety and fatigue are lemon balm, passionflower, and valerian.

- Low-dose (less than 1 mg) plant-based (not synthetic) melatonin, such as Herbatonin, can help with sleep initiation.

LIPID MANAGEMENT/HEART HEALTH

- Berberine has been recognized as capable of decreasing oxidative stress, LDL, triglycerides, and insulin resistance and improving mood.

- Maca has been shown to reduce blood pressure in menopausal women.

- Phytoestrogen extracts, including flax, hops, red clover, and soy foods, appear to have positive health effects on lipid concentrations and may reduce cardiovascular disease risk.

- Pycnogenol (pine bark extract) has been shown to reduce cardiovascular disease risk in menopause.

- Citrus Bergamot has been shown to reduce both overall as well as LDL cholesterol while increasing HDL cholesterol.

- Omega-3 fats, both foods and supplemental, have been shown to lower overall cholesterol.

LOW LIBIDO

- Herbs used specifically for low sex drive include horny goat weed, maca, and tribulus.

- Korean red ginseng may improve libido and mood.

- Saffron has been shown to improve libido and sexual function.

MOOD/ENERGY ISSUES

- Chasteberry (vitex) has been shown to significantly improve mood in menopause.

- Maca has been shown to improve mood.

- Pycnogenol (pine bark extract) has been shown to have a strong positive benefit on mood, anxiety, and fatigue in menopause.

- St. John's wort has been shown to improve mild to moderate depression and mood disorders related to menopause.

- Saffron has been shown to help with mood and lessen anxiety and depression.

- Bacopa monnieri has been shown to reduce anxiety and improve mood.

- Rhodiola has been shown to increase the levels of neurotransmitters which helps regulate mood.

OSTEOPOROSIS

- Omega-3 fats, both foods and supplemental, appear to help with bone density and mineralization.

- Some studies have shown that soy may help improve bone remodeling.

- Vitamin D3 combined with Vitamin K2 can help with bone growth and density.

Adaptogens for General Support

Adaptogens are herbal supplements derived primarily from mushrooms and plants. Adaptogens work by increasing or decreasing chemical reactions within your body to return it to a state of balance or homeostasis.

ASHWAGANDHA

- Ashwagandha is calming, supports energy, and may help reduce oxidative stress and improve sex drive.

- **Note:** Ashwagandha can interact with thyroid medications and raise T4 and T3 levels which can be problematic with hyperthyroidism. It can also worsen anhedonia, a condition in which one is unable to feel pleasure, which is common with depression and other mental health disorders.

HOLY BASIL (TULSI)

- Holy basil is a traditional and Ayurvedic herb used to help with fatigue and anxiety, with anti-inflammatory properties to support whole body wellness.

- Some studies suggest holy basil may even have cognitive benefits.

RHODIOLA

- This is used to lessen anxiety and can support the stress response, mental stamina, sleep, and mood.

- It is commonly used for longevity and healthy aging because of its impact on stress hormones and inflammation.

- It can also help with muscle recovery after exercise.

PEPTIDE THERAPY: AN EMERGING FRONTIER

One of the newer interventions being marketed to midlife women is an emerging therapy using peptides. Peptides are tiny proteins made up of short chains of amino acids that signal the cells in your body to perform in specific ways depending on the peptide used. Peptides are known as "secretagogues" because they stimulate the secretion of other chemicals or hormones. These therapies can take one of two forms: compounds that stimulate the pituitary gland to increase production and release of human growth hormone (these are also known as growth hormone–releasing peptides [GHRP] or growth hormone–releasing factors [GHRF]) *or* compounds that act outside growth hormone's actions by mimicking other molecules or hormones for their desired effects.

Peptide therapy involves the delivery of peptides via injections, creams, pills, or nasal sprays to stimulate the pituitary gland or other tissues. When taken as injections, peptides are usually administered subcutaneously either twice daily or once weekly. Peptide therapy via creams and pills is considered to have low efficacy due to poor bioavailability, and nasal sprays are newer with little testing for efficacy as of the time of writing.

The most commonly offered secretagogue peptides include CJC-1295, ipamorelin, BPC-157, and sermorelin. Other peptides to be aware of include bremelanotide PT-141 (brand name Vyleesi), semaglutide (Ozempic), and tirzepatide (Mounjaro). These named peptides only scratch the surface, however, as this is an emerging therapy and new peptides are constantly being brought to market.

From a pharmaceutical perspective, peptide therapy is a valid intervention for treatment of medical conditions such as obesity, diabetes, and chronic irritable bowel issues. That said, peptides are increasingly being sold to midlife women as fountains of youth to provide benefits such as anti-aging, belly fat and general weight reduction, skin tightening and cellulite elimination, muscle growth and body composition optimization, libido enhancement and sexual satisfaction, sleep enhancement, and general energy improvement. Although the promises are many, whether peptides can deliver their claimed benefits in nonmedical situations remains to be seen.

In addition to questions regarding their efficacy, peptides are not a simple or cost-effective intervention. Injectable peptides need to be kept refrigerated and oral peptides should not be taken around meals (because otherwise they will go into the digestive system as dietary protein). Although some claim that early results can be seen in as little as six weeks, most prescribers insist on a "loading" period of three to six months of uninterrupted use. Regardless of how long peptides are used, once stopped, their results most often disappear, with weight, skin wrinkles, and cellulite returning along with difficulty maintaining any achieved muscle, libido, sleep, and energy improvements.

Along with the potential for empty promises, peptides can also empty your wallet. Unless you have a medically required and insurance-approved prescription, peptides can carry an average monthly cost of up to $800 USD with annual costs topping out at around $15,000 USD. In addition to their expense, prolonged use of peptides may include some negative side effects. Some peptides can result in acromegaly, including enlarged feet, hands, and facial features; thickened and disfigured bones in the jaw, feet, and toes; and development of heart and kidney issues, diabetes, liver disease, joint pain, and fatigue. Other peptides can cause gastroparesis, a condition that affects the stomach muscles and prevents proper stomach emptying, and have been linked to thyroid cancer, among other conditions.

Given the incredible power of using lifestyle optimization, hormone therapy, and/or supplemental interventions, we have concerns about the push of peptide therapy on midlife women as if it is an answer to the symptoms and risks caused by hormone deprivation. While aesthetics are appealing, good health is and always has been the most important goal to work toward, so we see peptides as a distraction from which there is no good exit strategy.

While we believe that most women are able to take advantage of hormone therapy to protect their health, whether HRT is truly contraindicated for you or you simply are making the choice to not use it, we hope you can see that there are still powerful interventions to manage your quality of life as you age. In fact, the interventions of nutrition, movement, lifestyle, and supplemental support should be all midlife women's main priority. While we may all choose different paths, we are all on the same journey and these tools will ensure it is as healthy as possible!

PART FOUR

WHERE TO GO FROM HERE

CHAPTER FOURTEEN

THERE IS NO RIGHT OR WRONG, BUT INFORMED CONSENT MATTERS

HAVE YOU EVER EXPERIENCED the "red car" phenomenon—when you buy something (often a car) and, all of a sudden, you notice everyone else has the same car you do, even in the same color? You probably never paid attention to this car before you bought it, but now that you have one, everyone else seems to, too, right? This is how the topic of menopause seems today: It's everywhere all the time.

BEWARE OF THE MENOPAUSE GOLD RUSH

Whether it is a new podcast, book, online article, or social media post about menopause, a coach or practitioner who seemingly rebrands overnight into a menopause expert, or a celebrity or company pushing a menopause supplement or online mail-order hormone therapy–dispensing platform, the menopause bandwagon seems to be bursting at the seams. The hard truth is that with an estimated 1.2 billion women worldwide becoming postmenopausal by 2030, influencers, innovators, and investors are starting to pay attention to a market that has long been overlooked.

To be very frank, the topic of menopause has put dollar signs in their eyes—and all of us look like targets.

In addition to the profit opportunities, we believe another reason for this boom in menopause "awareness" is tied to the fact that 80 percent of medical residents admit they feel "barely comfortable" discussing or treating menopause. Enter influencers, venture capitalists, and anyone savvy enough to see an opportunity on the horizon.

This is where we say, **Beware:** You're no longer the consumer; you've become the product!

There is no argument that menopause is having a moment. As women who are deeply passionate about the subject of menopause and even more passionate about women receiving accurate information, we have to ask ourselves: Is this a good thing? Our answer is . . . yes and no.

Without a doubt, awareness and dialogue around menopause are good things. Midlife women are feeling heard and seen while finding the courage to speak up and seek help. Despite all the new attention, however, because of menopause's association with aging, there still exists an element of shame around it. Rather than enabling midlife women to celebrate a "well-lived" life and offering real solutions that allow us to age well, the menopause gold rush has stirred up an "anti-aging" movement with an intense focus on appearing younger.

Accordingly, most of the "solutions" being offered in the name of menopause are just skin deep (pun intended!). We need to shift the focus to how profoundly menopause and hormone loss change women's lives. It is time to start discussing—and sharing—the physiology of what is happening while creating a new standard of care that preserves women's healthspan. No matter how well marketed, shiny objects that address *only* symptoms and appearance are distraction rather than solutions.

We will just come out and say it: We are skeptical as to whether this (what feels like sudden) increase in menopause awareness will lead to deeper discussions on women's hormone needs. Why? Take one look at the profile of some of the more recent menopause products brought to market:

- An FDA-approved combination of bioidentical estradiol and progesterone; sounds great except that these are oral capsules in one-size-fits-all doses.

- An FDA-approved transdermal patch containing bioidentical estradiol (great!) with a progestin (an endocrine-disrupting synthetic progestogen—*not* great).

- Proprietary blends of herbal supplements promising "balance" (our hormones are never balanced, they fluctuate) to focus on symptoms (ignoring the deeper issues) with little to no identification of ingredient quality and quantity (code for including poor forms and synthetics) while also pitched as "safer" than HRT (HRT is not "unsafe"—and what is safe about keeping women deprived of hormones?), all while charging predatory pricing frequently via subscription models.

- Countless telemedicine platforms created by tech entrepreneurs using online questionnaires to offer mail-order hormones and other "solutions" (oral estradiol, Bi-Est, low doses of estrogen only, and poor-quality supplements) with no testing and lab data and creating no substantive doctor-patient relationship for monitoring.

- Menopause awareness–focused beauty companies with celebrity figureheads marketing consumer products for skin, hair, nails, and more, focusing women on their appearance as if it is a barometer of health (while ignoring or distracting them from the real imperatives underlying hormone deprivation).

Now, contrast those offerings with what you have learned throughout this book with regard to physiology and hormones, and ask yourself whether any of these accomplishes the goal of improving women's healthspan. They do not.

Menopause can be an amazing time in a woman's life but, from a health perspective, there is nothing about menopause that makes women healthier. For this reason, we celebrate and cheer all of the increased awareness around it. However, to the distraction of ineffective products and predatory companies attempting to catch your attention (and money), we give a big thumbs down. Throwing shiny objects at menopausal women and isolating the discussion to symptom relief is a huge disservice. Women need to be given a deep education about menopause to gain true fluency on what is happening to our physiology and the drastic changes that will eventually come. You now know better so you can do better—and we all should demand better.

YOU ARE AN INDIVIDUAL, SO STOP COMPARING WITH YOUR FRIENDS

One overlooked problem with all of the "new" talk around menopause is that there is a sort of implied message that we all experience the same thing. Although it is true that all women will have ovarian senescence leading to hormone deprivation, the experience of this progression and its aftermath are very individual. Think of menopause as similar to childbirth: You don't hear about women who have an easy transition, but you do hear about women who have a challenging, difficult time. In addition, the uncertainty about the signs, symptoms, and timing of menopause can truly shake our steadiness in midlife. Add to this list that our individual metabolic health going into the transition can be a significantly confounding variable and none of our menopause experiences will be the same.

Unfortunately, too many women will assess their own experience based on that of their friends, sisters, or mothers, and if it does not seem "as bad," then they determine there is nothing to discuss and no cause for attention. Similarly, if it is a worse experience or just markedly different, such as suddenly having high cholesterol and anxiety, then the conclusion is often that it may not be hormones at all and nonhormone therapeutic interventions such as statins or SSRIs are pursued instead.

Essentially, comparing your menopause transition with that of others often results in a missed opportunity to consider hormone therapy to address the true root cause of the changes and symptoms occurring. Thus, you expose yourself to increased disease risk as well as unintentional side effects from pharmaceuticals. In addition, there is a mental toll from your perceptions of having things better (as in you should not be complaining or concerned because it is not "as bad as" someone else's), worse (worrying something else could be wrong with you!), or just different from those around you.

Midlife and natural hormone changes can be very isolating at a time when we desperately need each other, and while it may be tempting to compare the nitty-gritty details of your journey with those of others, try to resist doing so and focus instead on the shared privilege of aging. With age comes a greater sense of acceptance of self and others, a desire for connection and the ability (and means) to create it, and personal knowledge to help make smart decisions. Sadly, not every woman will live long enough to have natural menopause and experience this phase of life, but if you are one of the lucky ones, choosing to focus on the wisdom, empathy, gratitude, and experiences that have enriched your life can be incredibly impactful—not only on your menopause experience but also on your overall healthspan.

MENOPAUSE MAY BE HAVING ITS MOMENT, BUT YOU ARE THE STAR

The menopause gold rush has, without a doubt, thrown menopause into the spotlight. Although this is partially a good thing, let's not overlook who really matters in this—you. Undeniably, hormone therapy is magic, but it is not a magic pill. You hold the cards for some of the most impactful menopause interventions to protect your healthspan: nutrition, movement, lifestyle, stress management, and community, upon which hormone therapy should be layered, when possible.

Finding a good HRT provider is not just about finding any provider willing to give you HRT. In fact, we say that you actually *should not* start your HRT journey with the provider—start with choosing what type of HRT you want to meet your goals, then find a provider aligned with you. Your goals should never be altered to meet whatever pleases your provider.

Informed consent is essential to personal autonomy when it comes to decisions about health. When health care providers are unable to effectively communicate with you about the true imperatives of the menopausal transition and hormone deprivation, let alone the options you have to address it, they are failing you. There is no right or wrong choice, only what is best for you. Yet, too many women are being denied the information they need to give informed consent when it comes to choosing or rejecting hormone therapy as well as how important nutrition and lifestyle are in midlife and beyond. This is not okay and this must change.

Here are just a few tips to recognize when a provider is not providing informed consent:

- They offer nonhormonal therapies (statins, SSRIs, sleep medications, bisphosphonates) as the first approach

- They offer birth control pills or pellets as HRT

- They tell you that *bioidentical* is "just a marketing term"

- They are critical of compounding pharmacies

- They tell you that hormones, especially estrogen, cause cancer

- They dismiss you as too old or too young

- They tell you that your grandmother's cancer makes you ineligible

- They tell you that labs and testing are unnecessary

For detailed steps on choosing the right HRT for you and finding a good HRT provider, see appendix E (page 182) and appendix F (page 184). Remember, when it comes to dealing with the imperatives of hormone deficiency due to menopause, this is your body, your choice, and your journey. Self-advocacy is your way to better health!

FINAL THOUGHTS

French physician Charles-Pierre-Louis De Gardanne coined the term *menopause* in the 1820s. He gets credit for calling attention to the change in a woman's hormonal and reproductive status and yet was widely criticized for emphasizing that this "critical time" was an inevitable entry into disease and decline. Given what we now know about the relationship of sex hormones to women's whole body health—cardiovascular health, cognitive function, bone health, the genitourinary system, and so much more—he was not wrong.

As we stated in the introduction, we wrote this book and have committed ourselves to educating women because we believe women have been misled about this crucial period of life and, because of it, have lost agency over their health. If you have read this far, you now have the insight and clarity needed to navigate the menopausal transition today and in the years ahead. Start slowly with daily intentional choices around nutrition and movement. Optimize your metabolic health and gut microbiome. Incorporate stress management techniques and prioritize rest and recovery. Seek testing to understand what might need attention in your body for better health. Evaluate your "community" and audit it so you are in the company of those who share your goals and passions. If you need or want more support, assemble a team of providers—health coaches, nutritionists, therapists, trainers, and other practitioners—who will help you carry out what you have learned. To that end, we would love to continue helping you as well!

We work with women around the globe dealing with hormone deficiency from a variety of causes. Our transformative program is built around an all-in-one method that pulls together resources such as lab-based testing and specialized instruction, comprehensive personal health assessments, one-on-one private contact, live interactive group coaching, and a private online community. This method gives us all a clear picture of you so we can focus on analyzing and addressing your unique needs. In return, you can expect a clear understanding of your unique health picture, with individualized guidance on midlife nutrition, exercise, and lifestyle modifications. We also provide targeted supplement support, hormone therapy insight, and, should you choose to purchase hormone therapy, for US and Canadian women, an HRT provider referral, or for international women, an

HRT advocate. You can find out more about our work at our website, WiseandWell.me, or take advantage of the free, education-forward resources and information we provide on Instagram at https://www.instagram.com/wise_and_well.

Every day is a new opportunity to put things into practice, with progress being the goal, not perfection. Know that this is an incredibly fulfilling time and, whether your menopause happened naturally or prematurely, you are poised to live an intentional, healthy, and thriving life. We wish you well and urge you to enjoy the journey!

OXIDATIVE PRIORITY

A Key Concept to Understand

OXIDATIVE PRIORITY IS A SORT OF DECISION TREE that the body uses to prioritize the order in which it will process the foods (fuels) you eat. This priority is directly based on how much of each fuel type you can store. When we are between meals, sleeping, or fasting (or any other unfed state), our bodies run on the fuels circulating in our blood or stored in our tissues. Once we eat something, however, the body stops relying on these internal fuels (as in, it stops burning fat) and, instead, uses the fuel coming in from the food.

With the goal of preventing an oversupply of fuel in the blood, your body chooses to either use or store the fuel before returning to homeostasis. Which source of fuel gets used first is determined by its place in the oxidative priority decision tree. Foods with higher priority will be processed before foods with lower priority, and if there is an oversupply, fuels of lower priority get stored. This means that to lose stored fat or to keep a steady weight, you must feed the body in a way that honors this oxidative priority:

1 Alcohol
2 Exogenous ketones
3 Protein
4 Carbohydrates
5 Fats

Let's say you have a lovely glass of wine with a meal of steak, sweet potatoes, and some sliced avocado. Although these are nutrient-dense whole foods, they may still hijack your goal of losing weight due to your body's priority for using the different fuels on your plate. To understand why, we need to examine the tree of priorities:

1 **Alcohol:** Like it or not, anytime you consume alcohol, your body will always choose it as a fuel first. Why? Because there is no storage for it and levels too high in the blood result in death. Only once the body burns off all the fuel from whatever alcohol you have consumed will it turn to burning other

fuels. This means that whenever you have a drink while eating, your body will end up storing most of the food while it deals with the alcohol. This is one reason alcohol can be so detrimental to fat loss.

2 **Exogenous ketones:** Although exogenous ketones aren't part of our hypothetical steak meal, once your body digests and burns alcohol, they are the next fuel source to be used. Exogenous ketones are supplements used to push the body into ketosis. Like alcohol, there is no storage capacity for exogenous ketones, and using them prevents your body from using other fuels. This is why having a cup of "bulletproof" coffee with MCT oil in the morning is actually breaking your fast: By consuming exogenous ketones, you are providing a preferential fuel to your body that triggers your metabolism and gets used before making your body use any stored fuel (fat) via fasting. Like alcohol, exogenous ketones are not biologically necessary and your body makes all the ketones you need when you are fat adapted, meaning your body will begin to burn body fat and dietary fat equally well and weight maintenance will be effortless.

3 **Protein:** The next fuel priority is protein, but protein is different from other fuels. Not only do we have a very limited amount of storage capacity for protein, but it also takes significantly more energy to turn protein into fuel (the "thermic effect" we discussed in chapter 5). For this reason, protein is only used as a fuel when there aren't other fuels (such as alcohol, carbs, or fat) present. If you are lean without a lot of fat storage and you do not oversupply your body with fat and carbs, your

body will meet your energy needs by turning protein into the fuel glucose through a process called *gluconeogenesis*. (This is an "as needed" process. Protein not needed as fuel is stored to its capacity or used for the immune system and to combat inflammation, and will then be excreted by the body. Excess protein does not end up as unneeded glucose! For most people, protein will be used primarily for muscle protein synthesis to build and repair lean tissues.) Protein is also biologically necessary, as our bodies are constantly turning over tissues and need a constant supply of amino acids to fuel this turnover.

4 **Carbohydrates:** Next are carbohydrates, and make note: We are not just talking about bagels and pastas, but any food that is primarily a carbohydrate, which breaks down into glucose. Carbs require the highest amount of insulin to be utilized and are not very satiating; some even leave you hungry when eaten in excess. The body processes carbs as the fuel glucose and then converts excess to glycogen, for which it has a moderate storage capacity (about 2,000 calories) in the liver and muscles. Although we can store carbs as glycogen in muscle, it is locked there and only really used in intense workouts like sprints or long episodes of exercise of at least ninety minutes or more in length. This means that a vigorous walk for an hour will not tap into this glycogen. That leaves only your liver for glycogen storage, but that capacity is around 100 grams of glucose. Excess glucose beyond storage capacity or needs gets turned into and stored as . . . fat. In addition, carbs are not biologically needed because your body can

make all the glucose it needs from stored fat (glycerol) or protein (via gluconeogenesis) once you are fat adapted.

5 **Fat:** The last priority in your body's fuel-processing decision tree is fat. Theoretically, we have unlimited storage space for fat. Although dietary fat can be used as fuel, more often than not it gets stored because (as we've just seen) other fuels take priority. Also, because fat requires the smallest amount of insulin to be processed, even just a small amount will break any fast and stop your body from burning its own fat. What fat has over carbs is that it is biologically essential and, calorie for calorie, is moderately satiating. While fat is needed to make hormones, absorb certain vitamins (A, D, E, and K), and facilitate cellular function, dietary fat will be used before any stored body fat as fuel. Thus, if you need or want to lose fat on your body, consider that stored fat as a fuel source rather than focusing on an independent dietary fat macro goal.

How to Use Oxidative Priority for Fat Loss

Now that you understand the body's oxidative priority, you are probably wondering what this means for losing fat. That's easy: Eliminate unnecessary fuels and keep dietary fat moderate enough to allow your body to focus on using its own (stored) fat for fuel. More specifically:

- Avoid alcohol and exogenous ketones.

- Get optimal protein to build and maintain lean mass (about 1 gram per pound [455 g] of desired body weight per day, distributed evenly throughout the day).

- Limit overall carbs according to your needs and goals.

- Reduce dietary fat just enough to force your body to use stored body fat as fuel (after protein, eat fat to satiety and to keep cravings and hunger at bay, but not to reach a goal or percentage).

When you meet your protein and carbohydrate goals and keep fat intake moderate for long enough (four to six weeks for most people), you will become and stay fat adapted.

CURRENT MARKET OPTIONS OFFERED AS HORMONE THERAPY

Injections

- **Estrogen Only**
  - ◆ Bioidentical: Note that Valerate and Cypionate are "esters" that are bound to estradiol to give it a longer lifetime in the blood. With esters, the hormone gets into the blood slowly over time, creating more even hormone levels (and reducing symptoms from hormone level changes). Some will argue that the presence of the esters make these estradiol injections nonbioidentical, but studies have shown that the body naturally decouples the esters from the hormone and only bioidentical 17-beta estradiol is the result.
    - » *Compounded: Estradiol Valerate/Cypionate*
    - » *Commercial: Delestrogen, Depo-Estradiol*
  - ◆ Nonbioidentical
    - » *Commercial: Premarin IV*

- **Progestogen Only**
  - ◆ Bioidentical
    - » *Commercial: Progesterone*
  - ◆ Nonbioidentical
    - » *Commercial: Makena*

- **Testosterone Only:** Intended only for male testosterone replacement therapy, these shots should never be used in women.

IUD

- **Progestogen** (levonorgestrel)
  - ◆ Nonbioidentical
    - » *Commercial: Kyleena, Liletta, Mirena, Skyla*

- **Copper Coil/Hormone-Acting**
  - ◆ Nonbioidentical
    - » *Commercial: Paraguard*

Low-Dose Birth Control Pills

- **Estrogen** (ethinyl estradiol and norethindrone)
  - Nonbioidentical
    - » *Commercial: (Lo)Estrin 1/20*
    - » *Estrogen plus Progestogen (Ethinylestradiol/ Levonorgestrel)*
  - Nonbioidentical
    - » *Commercial: Alesse*

Oral Pills

- **Oral Estrogens**
  - Bioidentical
    - » *Compounded: Estradiol, Estriol, Bi-Est, Tri-Est*
    - » *Commercial: Estrace*
  - Nonbioidentical
    - » *Commercial: Menest, Premarin*

- **Oral Progestogens**
  - Bioidentical (Progesterone)
    - » *Compounded: Progesterone*
    - » *Commercial: Prometrium*
  - Nonbioidentical (Progestins)
    - » *Commercial: Aygestin and Provera*

- **Oral Combined Estrogen plus Progestogens**
  - Bioidentical
    - » *Compounded: E2+P, E3+P, Bi-Est+P, Tri-Est+P*
    - » *Commercial: Bijuva (E2+P)*
  - Nonbioidentical (Synthetic Estrogens plus Progestins)
    - » *Commercial: Activella, Angeliq, FemHRT, Mimvey, Prefest, Premphase, Prempro*

- **Oral Testosterone**
  - Bioidentical
    - » *Compounded: Testosterone*
  - Nonbioidentical
    - » *Compounded: Methyltestosterone*

- **Oral Combined Testosterone plus Estrogen**
  - Nonbioidentical
    - » *Commercial: Covaryx*

Patches

- **Estrogen Only**
  - Bioidentical
    - » *Commercial: Alora, Climara, Menostar, Mini-velle, Vivelle Dot*

- **Estrogen plus Progestins**
  - Nonbioidentical
    - » *Commercial: Climara Pro, Combi Patch*

Pellets

- **Bioidentical**
  - Compounded: Estrogen, Testosterone, Estrogen and Testosterone together
  - Commercial: BioTe, EvexiPel, SottoPelle

Troches/Lozenges

- **Bioidentical**
  - Compounded: Estrogen, Progesterone, Testosterone

Topical Systemic Creams/Gels

- **Estrogen Only**
  - ◆ Bioidentical
    - » *Compounded: E2, E3, Bi-Est, Tri-Est*
    - » *Commercial: Divigel, Elestrin, Estrogel, Evamist*

- **Progesterone Only**
  - ◆ Bioidentical
    - » *Compounded: Progesterone*

- **Combined Estrogen plus Progesterone**
  - ◆ Bioidentical
    - » *Compounded: E2/E3/Bi-Est/Tri-Est plus Progesterone*

- **Testosterone Only**
  - ◆ Bioidentical
    - » *Compounded: Testosterone*

Vaginal Applications

- **Estrogens**
  - ◆ Bioidentical
    - » *Compounded: Estradiol, Estriol*
    - » *Commercial: Estrace, Estring, Imvexxy, Vagifem*
  - ◆ Nonbioidentical
    - » *Commercial: Femring, Premarin*

- **Progestogens**
  - ◆ Bioidentical
    - » *Compounded: Progesterone*
    - » *Commercial: Crinone/Prochieve, Endometrin*

- **DHEA**
  - ◆ Bioidentical
    - » *Compounded: DHEA*
    - » *Commercial: Intrarosa, Julva*

TESTS TO EVALUATE YOUR HORMONE THERAPY'S PERFORMANCE

ALTHOUGH CONVENTIONAL PHYSICIANS and physicians aligned with the North American Menopause Society will say that only symptom tracking is needed to determine the performance of hormone therapy, as discussed earlier, many women will normalize symptoms and so fail to report them as palpable or even problematic. In addition, many changes in our health do not have symptoms . . . until it is too late and the disease process has started (for example, we do not "feel" arterial stiffness or bone density loss). For these reasons, the only way to know whether your hormone therapy is achieving levels able to prevent or mitigate chronic disease processes is to test. Similarly, checking how your body is metabolizing and detoxing your hormones can help ensure that they are being excreted in a healthy manner. Finally, although observing the quality of daily bowel movements is recommended, checking the diversity and robustness of your microbiome bacterial profile through testing is recommended.

If your hormone therapy provider will not provide you with proper oversight testing, most of the tests listed here can be ordered via direct-to-consumer labs or from a functionally minded health practitioner who is trained in their interpretation.

HOW TO TRACK HORMONE SUFFICIENCY

The gold standard is to test hormones via blood serum, not blood spot, urine, or saliva. Testing is suggested every three months at initiation of hormone therapy and semiannually or annually thereafter.

- DHEA-S
- Estradiol
- FSH (follicle-stimulating hormone)
- Progesterone
- SHBG (sex hormone binding globulin)
- Testosterone

HOW TO MONITOR HORMONE METABOLISM

Testing is suggested every one to three years.

- Dried urine testing looking at detoxification and methylation
  - DUTCH Complete
  - HUMAP

HOW TO EVALUATE AND MONITOR YOUR GUT HEALTH

Testing is suggested as needed for digestive issues, or every one to three years.

- Stool tests for microbiome analysis
  - BiomeFx
  - GI360
  - GIMAP

TESTS TO EVALUATE YOUR METABOLIC HEALTH

ALTHOUGH IT WOULD BE IDEAL if we could assume that we are metabolically healthy based simply on something like our scale weight, the reality is that it is too simple to be "skinny" and unhealthy as well as possible to carry a little excess weight and still be quite healthy. For this reason, the only way to know whether your metabolic health is in check is to test various biomarkers in blood serum. Whether you enlist the help of your primary care doctor or self-monitor these things by using direct-to-consumer labs, following is a helpful list of basic markers to track annually, at a minimum, though more often is good, too! Having a functionally trained provider to interpret the results against optimal reference ranges (rather than lab-listed conventional ranges) is the best way to evaluate the status of your metabolic health.

Thyroid Status

- Free T4
- Free T3
- Reverse T3
- Thyroid antibodies
- TSH (thyroid-stimulating hormone)

Blood Sugar Regulation

- C-peptide
- Fasting insulin
- HOMA-IR or LP-IR
- Ratio of triglycerides to HDL-C
- Hemoglobin A1c

Inflammation Status

- Fibrinogen
- High sensitive C-reactive protein (hs-CRP)
- Homocysteine
- Sed rate (erythrocyte sedimentation rate, also known as ESR)
- Vitamin D

Oxidative Stress (often nutrient issues)

- B_{12} plus Folate
- CBC (complete blood count)
- CMP (comprehensive metabolic panel)
- Complete iron panel (ferritin, iron, iron saturation percentage, TIBC)
- GGT
- Magnesium
- Uric acid

Lipids: Quality and Quantity

- Apolipoprotein assessment
- Fractionated lipid panel with particles or NMR LipoProtein profile
- Lipoprotein(a) or Lp(a)

Other: Physical Markers

- 6-minute walk test
- 30-second sit to stand test
- Balance tests
- Blood pressure
- Grip strength (such as via a straight arm hang test)
- Waist-to-hip ratio (WHR)

HRT DECISION TREE

WHETHER PERIMENOPAUSAL or postmenopausal, do you want to start HRT? If yes, follow the decision tree.

- Do you have any contraindications (as explained in chapter 13)?
    - **Yes:** Determine whether a specialist is needed (oncologist, hematologist) to provide a medical opinion on a risk-benefit profile of HRT for you
    - **No:** Proceed

- Is your metabolic health within safe zones (no significant insulin resistance, inflammation, obesity, severe dysbiosis)?
    - **Yes:** Proceed
    - **No:** Work on nutrition and lifestyle, with supplemental interventions, before proceeding

- What are your goals?
    - Symptom management
        - » *Low-dose, static HRT would be sufficient and easiest*
    - Disease protection
        - » *Physiologic HRT should be pursued*

- Are you many years (more than ten) post-menopausal?
    - **Yes:** Physiologic rhythmic HRT is ideal (for receptor regeneration)
    - **No:** Proceed pursuant to goals

- Is your uterus intact and are you willing to have a managed monthly bleed?
    - **Yes:** Any physiologic rhythmic or physiologic cycled HRT
    - **No:** Physiologic static continuous combined HRT

- Do you have any transference or other lifestyle/convenience concerns?
    - **Yes:** Physiologic rhythmic HRT using compounded oral rhythmic progesterone and estradiol injections
    - **No:** Any physiologic rhythmic regimen

- Do you have significant sleep issues?
    - **Yes:** Physiologic rhythmic HRT with compounded oral rhythmic progesterone
    - **No:** Any physiologic rhythmic regimen

- Do you need treatment to be low cost or covered by insurance?
  - **Yes:** Physiologic with estradiol injections and oral Prometrium
  - **No:** Any form desired

Key to Terms

Physiologic (premenopausal levels of hormones)
- *Estradiol:* Compounded transdermal creams or commercial injections
- *Progesterone:* Compounded creams or pills or liquid

Rhythmic (dose varies over twenty-eight days)
- *Estradiol:* Compounded transdermal creams or commercial injections
- *Progesterone:* Compounded oral rhythmic capsules or liquid; NOT Prometrium

Static (same dose throughout twenty-eight days)
- *Estradiol:* Low-dose compounded cream or commercial patch
- *Progesterone:* Commercial Prometrium or compounded cream

Continuous (progesterone taken throughout twenty-eight days)
- *Estradiol plus progesterone*: Both taken every day with no breaks or dose variation

Cycled (progesterone taken only two weeks of the twenty-eight days)
- *Estradiol* taken every day *but* progesterone taken only two weeks on/two weeks off

Low Dose (enough to alleviate most symptoms but not provide disease protection)
- *Estradiol:* Compounded cream less than or equal to 1 mg/ml daily *or* commercial patch
- *Progesterone:* Oral capsules less than 100 mg

WISE & WELL GUIDE TO FINDING AN HRT PRACTITIONER

Conventional providers: The aim of hormone therapy is to prevent or improve complaints and symptoms caused by estrogen deficiency.

Physiologic providers: The primary goal of hormone therapy is to restore a hormonal environment as close to the natural, premenopausal state as possible to protect and improve long-term health risk.

Women are very different from one another. Our hormone levels during perimenopause and at menopause are as unique as our brain waves and fingerprints. Not only do we each have a unique genetic distribution of hormones and their receptors, but we also live, eat, drink, and move differently, which affects these things as well. Accordingly, each of us will respond differently to any given dose, route of delivery, and combination of hormones. For this reason, hormone therapy must be individually designed for maximum well-being and maintained for efficacy by monitoring hormone levels. This involves working with a seasoned provider who understands hormonal nuances, takes your hormone history into account, tests your lab values, and listens to your comments on how you feel. This provider not only tests your baseline levels but also commits to monitoring and tweaking things as needed because 1) even when a test appears "normal," how you feel is equally important and 2) we can feel well but have suboptimal hormone levels that fail to protect us from disease processes.

Maximizing the value of hormone therapy requires that doctors have a real appreciation of the way these hormones are metabolized and how much the body actually needs and can safely handle at any one time. Using too little may yield unsatisfactory results, whereas using too much may carry unacceptable risks. In this regard, what often gets lost in translation between symptom suppression and health optimization is giving any serious attention to the dose, timing, route of administration, and metabolic processing of these hormones.

If hormone therapy has any disadvantages, it is that it asks women to do more than just pop a pill every morning. It also requires doctors to monitor their patients' doses and hormone levels and to make sure the hormones are safely metabolized.

The proper use of hormone therapy demands:

- The correct mix of human bioidentical hormones
- The optimal physiologic amount of each hormone
- Taking hormones by the safest, most natural route
- Approximating the natural timing of hormone rhythms
- Close monitoring of the levels of hormones and their metabolites for safety

HOW DO YOU FIND A PROVIDER?

Many times, women think they can go to their gynecologist or primary care physician to manage their hormone therapy, but this is often not the case unless the doctor specializes in hormones and menopause. After reading this book, you will likely know more about hormone therapy than many gynecologists and other medical providers. Sad, but true. Although we need a competent, compassionate, licensed practitioner to manage our hormone therapy, please realize that just because someone is able (a.k.a. licensed) to write a prescription for hormones does not mean they should.

Before seeking out a practitioner:

1 Reread chapters 10 through 13 for fluency.

2 Review appendix E, HRT Decision Tree (page 182).

3 Start to form an idea about which method of delivery (creams/gels, patch, injections, etc.) will be good for you based on your lifestyle.

4 Research hormone therapy providers in your area; consider finding a local compounding pharmacy near you and asking which providers work with them who could provide hormone therapy that aligns with your goals.

   a Consider referrals from like-minded health coaches and/or trusted advisors who specialize in hormone therapy education.

   b Providers who label themselves as "ACOG" or "NAMS" or similar affiliations most often are providers of low-dose, static continuous hormones with the goal of symptom suppression.

   c Providers marketing themselves as "anti-aging" medicine providers *may* be in alignment with your goals, but interviewing them is key, as many see pellets as acceptable hormone therapy.

   d Note: Unfortunately, the title "Functional Medicine" or "IFM" by a provider's name does not give insight into their hormone therapy training, education, or expertise.

Interview the provider or their staff by asking these questions:

1 What is your stance on monitoring thyroid health while I am on HRT? Is this something you will do on an ongoing basis?

   Wise & Well thoughts: We believe that your HRT doctor should be willing and able to track your thyroid health and prescribe and adjust medication as needed. If they are unable or unwilling to do so, we suggest you keep going until you find someone who will manage both your HRT and your thyroid, whether or not you need medicine. The truth is, even if you don't need thyroid medicine now, you may need it at some point and you want to track this.

2 Do you have a preferred method of HRT? Do you deviate from your preferred method as needed?

   Wise & Well thoughts: If pellet therapy is the provider's preferred method, be wary. Please review the details in chapter 12 to understand why we say this. Also, be wary if they only offer Bi-Est or vaginal estrogens, as this seems to indicate a reluctance to fully embrace hormone therapy to improve health and may indicate a "fear" of estrogen. Similarly, offering you testosterone first, progesterone only long-term, or any "multihormone cocktails," whether cream or pellet, is a sign you should seek a different provider.

3 How often do I need to see you?

   Wise & Well thoughts: We believe that most women will need more oversight from their practitioner in the first year or two. This likely means two to four visits in each of years one and two after starting hormone therapy. If the response is that they will see you annually, you will not be getting the oversight needed to make sure that your hormone therapy is working optimally.

4 How often can I expect my HRT to be adjusted and what do you base the adjustments on?

   Wise & Well thoughts: The response from your practitioner should be: "Symptoms and lab work is what I base adjustments on."

5 How often am I expected to get lab work?

   Wise & Well thoughts: This can be anywhere from two to four times per year.

6 What are your fees and what do they include?

   Wise & Well thoughts: We do not really have any particular thoughts here except to say that there are doctors who charge an annual concierge fee and those who charge per visit. Likewise, some may include the cost of labs and some may not. Finally, although rare, some may even include the cost of the hormones themselves. It is important to ask these things up front so there are no surprises, and you can calculate the additional related costs of your hormone therapy (labs, prescriptions, etc.).

7 How do I communicate with you between visits, especially if there are issues or I have questions?

Wise & Well thoughts: Ideally, a hormone provider will have, at the very least, office staff members dedicated to being available to patients as needed, within reason. However, many have adopted virtual platforms and portals that foster communication via encrypted direct messaging, with options to schedule interim visits when necessary.

REFERENCES

PART I: HORMONES AND WOMEN'S HEALTH

Chapter One: Menopause Myths Are Affecting Women's Health

Against Violence and Abuse Project. Menopause and domestic abuse: early findings from AVA's Stuck in the Middle with You Project. October 18, 2021.

Allred C. Gray divorce rate in the U.S.: geographic variation, 2017. Bowling Green State University, National Center for Family & Marriage Research (NCFMR). Family Profile No. 20, 2019.

Brown SL, Lin IF. The gray divorce revolution: rising divorce among middle-aged and older adults, 1990–2010. J Gerontol B Psychol Sci Soc Sci. 2012 Nov;67(6):731–41. doi:10.1093/geronb/gbs089. Epub 2012 Oct 9. PMID: 23052366; PMCID: PMC3478728.

Brown SL, Wright MR. Divorce attitudes among older adults: two decades of change. J Fam Issues. 2019 Jun;40(8):1018–1037. doi:10.1177/0192513X19832936. Epub 2019 Feb 27. PMID: 31749514; PMCID: PMC6867609.

Farrelly C. Longevity science and women's health and well-being. J Popul Ageing. 2023 Jan 30:1–20. doi:10.1007/s12062-023-09411-y. Epub ahead of print. PMID: 36741335; PMCID: PMC9885070.

Faubion SS, Enders F, Hedges MS, Chaudhry R, Kling JM, Shufelt CL, Saadedine M, Mara K, Griffin JM, Kapoor E. Impact of menopause symptoms on women in the workplace. Mayo Clin Proc. 2023 Jun;98(6):833–45. doi:10.1016/j.mayocp.2023.02.025. Epub 2023 Apr 26. PMID: 37115119.

Garmany A, Yamada S, Terzic A. Longevity leap: mind the healthspan gap. npj Regen Med. 2021;6:57. https://doi.org/10.1038/s41536-021-00169-5

Grand View Research. Menopause Market Size, Share & Trends Analysis Report by Treatment (Dietary Supplements, OTC Pharma Products), by Region (North America, Europe, APAC, Latin America, MEA), and Segment Forecasts, 2023–2030. Report ID: GVR-4-68039-434-2.

Hägg S, Jylhävä J. Sex differences in biological aging with a focus on human studies. eLife, 2021. 10:e63425. https://doi.org/10.7554/eLife.63425.

Hill K. The demography of menopause. Maturitas. 1996 Mar;23(2):113–27. doi:10.1016/0378-5122(95)00968-x. PMID: 8735350.

Kachel AF, Premo LS, Hublin JJ. Grandmothering and natural selection. Proc Biol Sci. 2011 Feb 7;278(1704):384–91. doi:10.1098/rspb.2010.1247. Epub 2010 Aug 25. PMID: 20739319; PMCID: PMC3013409.

Levin S, Van Haren PC. "70s Are the New 50s: How Grey Divorce Differs from a Typical Divorce." American Bar Association Journal, March 9, 2022.

MacNee W, Rabinovich RA, Choudhury G. Ageing and the border between health and disease. Eur Respir J. 2014 Nov;44(5):1332–52. doi:10.1183/09031936.00134014. Epub 2014 Oct 16. PMID: 25323246.

Ortiz-Ospina E, Beltekian D. Why do women live longer than men? Our World in Data. August 14, 2018.

Park A. Menopause Makes Your Body Age Faster. Time. July 25, 2016. Retrieved online.

Sarrel PM, Njike VY, Vinante V, Katz DL. The mortality toll of estrogen avoidance: an analysis of excess deaths among hysterectomized women aged 50 to 59 years. Am J Public Health. 2013 Sep;103(9):1583–88. doi:10.2105/AJPH.2013.301295. Epub 2013 Jul 18. PMID: 23865654; PMCID: PMC3780684.

Chapter Two: Female Hormones: Understanding the Changing Midlife Landscape

Ansere VA, Ali-Mondal S, Sathiaseelan R, Garcia DN, Isola JVV, Henseb JD, Saccon TD, Ocañas SR, Tooley KB, Stout MB, Schneider A, Freeman WM. Cellular hallmarks of aging emerge in the ovary prior to primordial follicle depletion. Mech Ageing Dev. 2021 Mar;194:111425. doi:10.1016/j.mad.2020.111425. Epub 2020 Dec 28. PMID: 33383072; PMCID: PMC8279026.

Cable JK, Grider MH. Physiology, Progesterone. [Updated 2022 May 8]. In: StatPearls [Internet]. Treasure Island (FL): StatPearls Publishing; 2022 Jan-. Available from: https://www.ncbi.nlm.nih.gov/books/NBK558960.

Campbell M, Jialal I. Physiology, Endocrine Hormones. [Updated 2022 Sep 26]. In: StatPearls [Internet]. Treasure Island (FL): StatPearls Publishing; 2022 Jan-. Available from: https://www.ncbi.nlm.nih.gov/books/NBK538498.

Cui J, Shen Y, Li R. Estrogen synthesis and signaling pathways during aging: from periphery to brain. Trends Mol Med. 2013 Mar;19(3):197–209. doi:10.1016/j.molmed.2012.12.007. Epub 2013 Jan 22. PMID: 23348042; PMCID: PMC3595330.

Harlow SD, Gass M, Hall JE, Lobo R, Maki P, Rebar RW, Sherman S, Sluss PM, de Villiers TJ; STRAW 10 Collaborative Group. Executive summary of the Stages of Reproductive Aging Workshop + 10: addressing the unfinished agenda of staging reproductive aging. Menopause. 2012 Apr;19(4):387–95. doi:10.1097/gme.0b013e31824d8f40. PMID: 22343510; PMCID: PMC3340903.

Menstrual Cycles as a Fifth Vital Sign. https://www.nichd.nih.gov/about/org/od/directors_corner/prev_updates/menstrual-cycles.

Nassar GN, Leslie SW. Physiology, Testosterone. [Updated 2022 Jan 4]. In: StatPearls [Internet]. Treasure Island (FL): StatPearls Publishing; 2022 Jan-. Available from: https://www.ncbi.nlm.nih.gov/books/NBK526128.

Nelson LR, Bulun SE. Estrogen production and action. J Am Acad Dermatol. 2001 Sep;45(3 Suppl):S116–24. doi:10.1067/mjd.2001.117432. PMID: 11511861.

Patel P, Abate N. Body fat distribution and insulin resistance. Nutrients. 2013 Jun 5;5(6):2019–27. doi:10.3390/nu5062019. PMID: 23739143; PMCID: PMC3725490.

Tebbens M, et al. The role of estrone in feminizing hormone treatment. J of Clin Endocrin & Metab. 2022 Feb;107(2): e458–e466. https://doi.org/10.1210/clinem/dgab741.

Yiallouris A, Tsioutis C, Agapidaki E, Zafeiri M, Agouridis AP, Ntourakis D, Johnson EO. Adrenal aging and its implications on stress responsiveness in humans. Front Endocrinol. 2019 Feb 7;10:54. doi:10.3389/fendo.2019.00054. PMID: 30792695; PMCID: PMC6374303.

Chapter Three: Female Hormones Beyond Fertility: Effects of Estrogen and Progesterone on Whole Body Health

Afsaneh B, Medea Lenz A, Labonte MJ, Lenz HJ. Molecular pathways: estrogen pathway in colorectal cancer. Clin Cancer Res. 2013 Nov;19(21):5842–48. https://doi.org/10.1158/1078-0432.CCR-13-0325.

Arruvito L, Giulianelli S, Flores AC, Paladino N, Barboza M, Lanari C, Fainboim L. NK cells expressing a progesterone receptor are susceptible to progesterone-induced apoptosis. J Immunol. 2008 Apr 15;180(8):5746–53. doi:10.4049/jimmunol.180.8.5746. PMID: 18390760.

Bader A, Sacrez J, Langer B, Sacrez A. Oestrogènes naturels et système cardio-vasculaire [Natural estrogens and the cardiovascular system]. J Gynecol Obstet Biol Reprod (Paris). 1996;25(3):233–37. French. PMID: 8767217.

Baker JM, Al-Nakkash L, Herbst-Kralovetz MM. Estrogen-gut microbiome axis: physiological and clinical implications. Maturitas. 2017 Sep;103:45–53. doi:10.1016/j.maturitas.2017.06.025. Epub 2017 Jun 23. PMID: 28778332.

Batra SC, Iosif LS. Progesterone receptors in the female urinary tract. J Urol 1987;138:130–34.

Baulieu E, Schumacher M. Progesterone as a neuroactive neurosteroid, with special reference to the effect of progesterone on myelination. Steroids. 2000 Oct-Nov; 65(10-11):605–12. doi:10.1016/s0039-128x(00)00173-2. PMID: 11108866.

Benedek G, Zhang J, Nguyen H, Kent G, Seifert HA, Davin S, Stauffer P, Vandenbark AA, Karstens L, Asquith M, Offner H. Estrogen protection against EAE modulates the microbiota and mucosal-associated regulatory cells. J Neuroimmunol. 2017 Sep 15;310:51–59. doi:10.1016/j.jneuroim.2017.06.007. Epub 2017 Jun 21. PMID: 28778445; PMCID: PMC5570519.

Berent-Spillson A, Briceno E, Pinsky A, Simmen A, Persad CC, Zubieta JK, Smith YR. Distinct cognitive effects of estrogen and progesterone in menopausal women. Psychoneuroendocrinology. 2015 Sep;59:25–36. doi:10.1016/j.psyneuen.2015.04.020. Epub 2015 May 14. PMID: 26010861; PMCID: PMC4490102.

Berger C, Qian Y, Chen X. The p53-estrogen receptor loop in cancer. Curr Mol Med. 2013 September;13(8):1229–40. doi:10.2174/15665240113139990065. PMID: 23865427; PMCID: PMC3780397.

Booth EA, Lucchesi BR. Estrogen-mediated protection in myocardial ischemia-reperfusion injury. Cardiovasc Toxicol. 2008 Fall;8(3):101–13. doi:10.1007/s12012-008-9022-2. Epub 2008 Aug 6. PMID: 18683081.

Borrás C, Gambini J, López-Grueso R, Pallardó FV, Viña J. Direct antioxidant and protective effect of estradiol on isolated mitochondria. Molecular Basis of Dis. 2010(1802)1:205–11.

Brown LM, Clegg DJ. Central effects of estradiol in the regulation of food intake, body weight, and adiposity. J Steroid Biochem Mol Biol. 2010 Oct;122(1–3):65–73. doi:10.1016/j.jsbmb.2009.12.005. Epub 2009 Dec 24. PMID: 20035866; PMCID: PMC2889220.

Chen KL, Madak-Erdogan Z. Estrogen and microbiota crosstalk: should we pay attention? Trends Endocrinol Metab. 2016 Nov;27(11):752–55. doi:10.1016/j.tem.2016.08.001. Epub 2016 Aug 20. PMID: 27553057.

Chen Q, Zhang W, Sadana N, et al. Estrogen receptors in pain modulation: cellular signaling. Biol Sex Differ. 2021;12:22. https://doi.org/10.1186/s13293-021-00364-5.

Chen TS, Doong ML, Chang FY, Lee SD, Wang PS. Effects of sex steroid hormones on gastric emptying and gastrointestinal transit in rats. Am J Physiol. 1995 Jan;268(1 Pt 1):G17–6. doi:10.1152/ajpgi.1995.268.1.G171. PMID: 7840200.

Ciesielska A, Kusiak A, Ossowska A, Grzybowska ME. Changes in the oral cavity in menopausal women: a narrative review. Int J Environ Res Public Health. 2021 Dec 27;19(1):253. doi:10.3390/ijerph19010253. PMID: 35010513; PMCID: PMC8750983.

Cutolo M, Smith V, Paolino S. Understanding immune effects of oestrogens to explain the reduced morbidity and mortality in female versus male COVID-19 patients: comparisons with autoimmunity and vaccination. Clin Exp Rheumatol. 2020 May-Jun;38(3):383–86. doi:10.55563/clinexprheumatol/qb05rr. Epub 2020 May 12. PMID: 32452350.

Di Martino V, Lebray P, Myers RP, Pannier E, Paradis V, Charlotte F, Moussalli J, Thabut D, Buffet C, Poynard T. Progression of liver fibrosis in women infected with hepatitis C: long-term benefit of estrogen exposure. Hepatology. 2004 Dec;40(6):1426–33. doi:10.1002/hep.20463. PMID: 15565616.

Ebbeling CB, Feldman HA, Klein GL, Wong JMW, Bielak L, Steltz SK, Luoto PK, Wolfe RR, Wong WW, Ludwig DS. Effects of a low carbohydrate diet on energy expenditure during weight loss maintenance: randomized trial. BMJ. 2018;363:k4583

Espinoza TR, Wright DW. The role of progesterone in traumatic brain injury. J Head Trauma Rehabil. 2011 Nov-Dec;26(6):497–99. doi:10.1097/HTR.0b013e31823088fa. PMID: 22088981; PMCID: PMC6025750.

Ferretti G, Felici A, Cognetti F. The protective side of progesterone. Breast Cancer Res. 2007;9(6):402. doi:10.1186/bcr1792. PMID: 18086325; PMCID: PMC2246175.

Fischer B, Gleason C, Asthana S. Effects of hormone therapy on cognition and mood. Fertil Steril. 2014 Apr;101(4):898–904. doi:10.1016/j.fertnstert.2014.02.025. PMID: 24680649; PMCID: PMC4330961.

Fishman J, Martucci CP. New Concepts of Estrogenic Activity: The Role of Metabolites in the Expression of Hormone Action. In Pasetto, N, Paoletti R, Ambrus JL. The Menopause and Postmenopause. 1980, 43–52. doi:10.1007/978-94-011-7230-1_5. ISBN 978-94-011-7232-5.

Freer G, Matteucci D. Influence of dendritic cells on viral pathogenicity. PLoS Pathog. 2009 Jul;5(7):e1000384. doi:10.1371/journal.ppat.1000384. Epub 2009 Jul 31. PMID: 19649323; PMCID: PMC2712770.

Gasco M, Shami S, Crook T. The p53 pathway in breast cancer. Breast Cancer Res. 2002;4(2):70–6. doi:10.1186/bcr426. Epub 2002 Feb 12. PMID: 11879567; PMCID: PMC138723.

Gupte AA, Pownall HJ, Hamilton DJ. Estrogen: an emerging regulator of insulin action and mitochondrial function. J Diabetes Res. 2015;2015:916585. doi:10.1155/2015/916585. Epub 2015 Mar 26. PMID: 25883987; PMCID: PMC4391691.

Guzman RC, Yang J, Rajkumar L, Thordarson G, Chen X, Nandi S. Hormonal prevention of breast cancer: mimicking the protective effect of pregnancy. Proc Natl Acad Sci U S A. 1999 Mar 2;96(5):2520–25. doi:10.1073/pnas.96.5.2520. PMID: 10051675; PMCID: PMC26817.

Hall OJ, Limjunyawong N, Vermillion MS, Robinson DP, Wohlgemuth N, Pekosz A, Mitzner W, Klein SL. Progesterone-based therapy protects against influenza by promoting lung repair and recovery in females. PLoS Pathog. 2016 Sep 15;12(9):e1005840. doi:10.1371/journal.ppat.1005840. PMID: 27631986; PMCID: PMC5025002.

Hara Y, Waters EM, McEwen BS, Morrison JH. Estrogen effects on cognitive and synaptic health over the lifecourse. Physiol Rev. 2015 Jul;95(3):785–807. doi:10.1152/physrev.00036.2014. PMID: 26109339; PMCID: PMC4491541.

Hirschberg AL. Sex hormones, appetite and eating behaviour in women. Maturitas. 2012 Mar;71(3):248–56. doi:10.1016/j.maturitas.2011.12.016. Epub 2012 Jan 26. PMID: 22281161.

Hoffmann M, Kleine-Weber H, Schroeder S, Krüger N, Herrler T, Erichsen S, Schiergens TS, Herrler G, Wu NH, Nitsche A, Müller MA, Drosten C, Pöhlmann S.

SARS-CoV-2 cell entry depends on ACE2 and TMPRSS2 and is blocked by a clinically proven protease inhibitor. Cell. 2020 Apr 16;181(2):271–80.e8. doi:10.1016/j.cell.2020.02.052. Epub 2020 Mar 5. PMID: 32142651; PMCID: PMC7102627.

Horvath G, Leser G, Karlsson L, Delle U. Estradiol regulates tumor growth by influencing p53 and bcl-2 expression in human endometrial adenocarcinomas grown in nude mice. In Vivo. 1996 Jul-Aug;10(4):411–16. PMID: 8839787.

Iosif S, Batra S, Ek A, et al. Oestrogens receptors in the human female lower urinary tract. Am J Obstet Gynaecol .1981;141:817–20.

Kamada M, Irahara M, Maegawa M, Yasui T, Yamano S, Yamada M, Tezuka M, Kasai Y, Deguchi K, Ohmoto Y, Aono T. B cell subsets in postmenopausal women and the effect of hormone replacement therapy. Maturitas. 2001 Jan 31;37(3):173–79. doi:10.1016/s0378-5122(00)00180-8. PMID: 11173179.

Kennelly R, Kavanagh DO, Hogan AM, Winter DC. Oestrogen and the colon: potential mechanisms for cancer prevention. Lancet Oncol. 2008 Apr;9(4):385–91. doi:10.1016/S1470-2045(08)70100-1. PMID: 18374292.

Khosla S, Oursler MJ, Monroe DG. Estrogen and the skeleton. Trends Endocrinol Metab. 2012 Nov;23(11):576–81. doi:10.1016/j.tem.2012.03.008. Epub 2012 May 16. PMID: 22595550; PMCID: PMC3424385.

Kim YJ, Soto M, Branigan GL, Rodgers K, Brinton RD. Association between menopausal hormone therapy and risk of neurodegenerative diseases: implications for precision hormone therapy. Alzheimer's Dement. 2021 May 13;7(1):e12174. doi:10.1002/trc2.12174. PMID: 34027024; PMCID: PMC8118114.

Klinge CM. Estrogenic control of mitochondrial function and biogenesis. J Cell Biochem. 2008 Dec 15;105(6):1342–51. doi:10.1002/jcb.21936. PMID: 18846505; PMCID: PMC2593138.

Kovats S. Estrogen receptors regulate innate immune cells and signaling pathways. Cell Immunol. 2015 Apr;294(2):63–69. doi:10.1016/j.cellimm.2015.01.018. Epub 2015 Feb 7. PMID: 25682174; PMCID: PMC4380804.

Kuhl H. Pharmacology of estrogens and progestogens: influence of different routes of administration (PDF). Climacteric. 2005 Aug;8:Suppl 1: 3–63. doi:10.1080/13697130500148875. PMID 16112947. S2CID 24616324.

Kwa M, Plottel CS, Blaser MJ, Adams S. The intestinal microbiome and estrogen receptor-positive female breast cancer. J Natl Cancer Inst. 2016 Apr 22;108(8):djw029. doi:10.1093/jnci/djw029. PMID: 27107051; PMCID: PMC5017946.

Lacasa D, Le Liepvre X, Ferre P, Dugail I. Progesterone stimulates adipocyte determination and differentiation 1/sterol regulatory element-binding protein 1c gene expression: potential mechanism for the lipogenic effect of progesterone in adipose tissue. J Biol Chem. 2001 Apr 13;276(15):11512–16. doi:10.1074/jbc.M008556200. Epub 2001 Jan 16. PMID: 11278421.

Lindblad M, Ye W, Rubio C, Lagergren J. Estrogen and risk of gastric cancer: a protective effect in a nationwide cohort study of patients with prostate cancer in Sweden. Cancer Epidemiol Biomarkers Prev. 2004 Dec;13(12):2203–7. PMID: 15598781.

Liu CY, Chen LB, Liu PY, Xie DP, Wang PS. Effects of progesterone on gastric emptying and intestinal transit in male rats. World J Gastroenterol. 2002 Apr;8(2):338–41. doi:10.3748/wjg.v8.i2.338. PMID: 11925620; PMCID: PMC4658379.

Marei HE, Althani A, Afifi N, et al. p53 signaling in cancer progression and therapy. Cancer Cell Int. 2021;21:703. https://doi.org/10.1186/s12935-021-02396-8.

Martin-Millan M, Almeida M, Ambrogini E, Han L, Zhao H, Weinstein RS, Jilka RL, O'Brien CA, Manolagas SC. The estrogen receptor-alpha in osteoclasts mediates the protective effects of estrogens on cancellous but not cortical bone. Mol Endocrinol. 2010 Feb;24(2):323–34. doi:10.1210/me.2009-0354. Epub 2010 Jan 6. PMID: 20053716; PMCID: PMC2817608.

McCarthy M, Raval AP. The peri-menopause in a woman's life: a systemic inflammatory phase that enables later neurodegenerative disease. J Neuroinflammation. 2020 Oct 23;17(1):317. doi:10.1186/s12974-020-01998-9. PMID: 33097048; PMCID: PMC7585188.

Mooga VP, et al. Estrogen and mitochondrial function in disease. Mitochondrial Dis, InTech, 2018 Aug. doi:10.5772/intechopen.73015.

Mozo J, Emre Y, Bouillaud F, Ricquier D, Criscuolo F. Thermoregulation: what role for UCPs in mammals and birds? Biosci Rep. 2005 Jun-Aug;25(3-4):227–49. doi:10.1007/s10540-005-2887-4. PMID: 16283555.

Nakamura T, Imai Y, Matsumoto T, Sato S, Takeuchi K, Igarashi K, Harada Y, Azuma Y, Krust A, Yamamoto Y, Nishina H, Takeda S, Takayanagi H, Metzger D, Kanno J, Takaoka K, Martin TJ, Chambon P, Kato S. Estrogen prevents bone loss via estrogen receptor alpha and induction of Fas ligand in osteoclasts. Cell. 2007 Sep 7;130(5):811–23. doi:10.1016/j.cell.2007.07.025. PMID: 17803905.

Pare G, Krust A, Karas RH, Dupont S, Aronovitz M, Chambon P, Mendelsohn ME. Estrogen receptor-alpha mediates the protective effects of estrogen against vascular injury. Circ Res. 2002 May 31;90(10):1087–92. doi:10.1161/01.res.0000021114.92282.fa. PMID: 12039798.

Parini P, Angelin B, Rudlin M. Importance of estrogen receptors in hepatic LDL receptor regulation. Arter, Thromb, and Vasc Biol. 1977;1):800–05.

Pfeffer CM, Singh ATK. Apoptosis: a target for anti-cancer therapy. Int J Mol Sci. 2018 Feb 2;19(2):448. doi:10.3390/ijms19020448. PMID: 29393886; PMCID: PMC5855670.

Rapkin AJ. Progesterone, GABA and mood disorders in women. Arch Women's Mental Health. 1999 Nov;2(3):0097–105. http://resolver.scholarsportal.info/resolve/14341816/v02i0003/0097_pgamdiw.xml.

Rogers A, Eastell R. Effects of estrogen therapy of post-menopausal women on cytokines measured in peripheral blood. J Bone Miner Res. 1998 Oct;13(10):1577–86. doi:10.1359/jbmr.1998.13.10.1577. PMID: 9783546.

Sasso CV, Santiano FE, Campo Verde Arboccó F, Zyla LE, Semino SN, Guerrero-Gimenez ME, Pistone Creydt V, López Fontana CM, Carón RW. Estradiol and progesterone regulate proliferation and apoptosis in colon cancer. Endocr Connect. 2019 Mar 1;8(3):217–29. doi:10.1530/EC-18-0374. PMID: 30738018; PMCID: PMC6391933.

Shi L, Feng Y, Lin H, Ma R, Cai X. Role of estrogen in hepatocellular carcinoma: is inflammation the key? J Transl Med. 2014 Apr 8;12:93. doi:10.1186/1479-5876-12-93. PMID: 24708807; PMCID: PMC3992128.

Shuster BZ, Depireux DA, Mong JA, Hertzano R. Sex differences in hearing: probing the role of estrogen signaling. J Acoust Soc Am. 2019 Jun;145(6):3656. doi:10.1121/1.5111870. PMID: 31255106; PMCID: PMC6588519.

Siow RC, Li FY, Rowlands DJ, de Winter P, Mann GE. Cardiovascular targets for estrogens and phytoestrogens: transcriptional regulation of nitric oxide synthase and antioxidant defense genes. Free Radic Biol Med. 2007 Apr 1;42(7):909–25. doi:10.1016/j.freeradbiomed.2007.01.004. Epub 2007 Jan 8. PMID: 17349919.

Stevenson S, Thornton J. Effect of estrogens on skin aging and the potential role of SERMs. Clin Interv Aging. 2007;2(3):283–97. doi:10.2147/cia.s798. PMID: 18044179; PMCID: PMC2685269.

Sullivan SD, Sarrel PM, Nelson LM. Hormone replacement therapy in young women with primary ovarian insufficiency and early menopause. Fertil Steril. 2016 Dec;106(7):1588–99. doi:10.1016/j.fertnstert.2016.09.046. PMID: 27912889; PMCID: PMC5137796.

Tagliaferri C, Salles J, Landrier JF, Giraudet C, Patrac V, Lebecque P, Davicco MJ, Chanet A, Pouyet C, Dhaussy A, Huertas A, Boirie Y, Wittrant Y. Coxam V, Walrand S. Increased body fat mass and tissue lipotoxicity associated with ovariectomy or high-fat diet differentially affects bone and skeletal muscle metabolism in rats. Eur J Nutr. 2015;54:1139–49.

Thomas P, Pang Y. Protective actions of progesterone in the cardiovascular system: potential role of membrane progesterone receptors (mPRs) in mediating rapid effects. Steroids. 2013 Jun;78(6):583–88. doi:10.1016/j.steroids.2013.01.003. Epub 2013 Jan 25. PMID: 23357432.

Thornton MJ. Estrogens and aging skin. Dermatoendocrinol. 2013 Apr 1;5(2):264–70. doi:10.4161/derm.23872. PMID: 24194966; PMCID: PMC3772914.

Twombly R. Estrogen's dual nature? Studies highlight effects on breast cancer. J Natl Cancer Inst. 2011 June 22;103 (12):920–21. doi:10.1093/jnci/djr233. PMID: 21693756.

Wald A, Van Thiel DH, Hoechstetter L, Gavaler JS, Egler KM, Verm R, Scott L, Lester R. Gastrointestinal transit: the effect of the menstrual cycle. Gastroenterology. 1981 Jun;80(6):1497–500. PMID: 7227774.

Walton C, Godsland IF, Proudler AJ, Wynn V, Stevenson JC. The effects of the menopause on insulin sensitivity, secretion and elimination in non-obese, healthy women. European J Clin Inv. 1993;23:466–73.

Webb P. 24-hour energy expenditure and the menstrual cycle. Am J Clin Nutr. 1986 Nov;44(5):614–19. doi:10.1093/ajcn/44.5.614. PMID: 3766447.

Yang S, Thiel KW, Leslie KK. Progesterone: the ultimate endometrial tumor suppressor. Trends Endocrinol Metab. 2011 Apr;22(4):145–52. doi:10.1016/j.tem.2011.01.005. Epub 2011 Feb 25. PMID: 21353793; PMCID: PMC4062362.

Chapter Four: Midlife Changes: Why Women Need to Take Charge Before the Signs and Symptoms Start

Abdi F, Mobedi H, Bayat F, Mosaffa N, Dolatian M, Ramezani Tehrani F. The effects of transdermal estrogen delivery on bone mineral density in postmenopausal women: a meta-analysis. Iran J Pharm Res. 2017 Winter;16(1):380–89. PMID: 28496491; PMCID: PMC5423263.

Albright F, Smith Ph, Richardson Am. Postmenopausal osteoporosis: its clinical features. JAMA. 1941;116(22):2465–74. doi:10.1001/jama.1941.02820220007002.

Anagnostis P, Athyros VG, Tziomalos K, Karagiannis A, Mikhailidis DP. Clinical review: the pathogenetic role of cortisol in the metabolic syndrome: a hypothesis. J Clin Endocrinol Metab. 2009 Aug;94(8):2692–701. doi:10.1210/jc.2009-0370. Epub 2009 May 26. PMID: 19470627.

Angelou K, Grigoriadis T, Diakosavvas M, Zacharakis D, Athanasiou S. The genitourinary syndrome of menopause: an overview of the recent data. Cureus. 2020 Apr 8;12(4):e7586. doi:10.7759/cureus.7586. PMID: 32399320; PMCID: PMC7212735.

Armstrong CM, Billimek AR, Allred KF, Sturino JM, Weeks BR, Allred CD. A novel shift in estrogen receptor expression occurs as estradiol suppresses inflammation-associated colon tumor formation. Endocr Relat Cancer. 2013 Jun 27;20(4):515–25. doi:10.1530/ERC-12-0308. PMID: 23702470.

Bado I, Nikolos F, Rajapaksa G, et al. Somatic loss of estrogen receptor beta and p53 synergize to induce breast tumorigenesis. BCR. 2017 Jul;19(1):79. DOI:10.1186/s13058-017-0872-z. PMID: 28673316; PMCID: PMC5494907.

Baker JM, Al-Nakkash L, Herbst-Kralovetz MM. Estrogen-gut microbiome axis: physiological and clinical implications. Maturitas. 2017 Sep;103:45–53. doi:10.1016/j.maturitas.2017.06.025. Epub 2017 Jun 23. PMID: 28778332.

Brincat M, Versi E, Moniz CF, et al. Skin collagen changes in postmenopausal women receiving different regimens of estrogen therapy. Obstet Gynecol. 1987 Jul;70(1):123–27. PMID: 3601260.

Brinton RD, Yao J, Yin F, Mack WJ, Cadenas E. Peri-menopause as a neurological transition state. Nat Rev Endocrinol. 2015 Jul;11(7):393–405. doi:10.1038/nrendo.2015.82. Epub 2015 May 26. PMID: 26007613; PMCID: PMC9934205.

Broz P, Dixit VM. Inflammasomes: mechanism of assembly, regulation and signalling. Nat Rev Immunol. 2016;16(7):407–20.

Caiazza F, Ryan EJ, Doherty G, Winter DC, Sheahan K. Estrogen receptors and their implications in colorectal carcinogenesis. Front Oncol. 2015 Feb 2;5:19. doi:10.3389/fonc.2015.00019. PMID: 25699240; PMCID: PMC4313613.

Campbell SE, Febbraio MA. Effect of the ovarian hormones on GLUT4 expression and contraction-stimulated glucose uptake. Am J Physiol Endocrinol Metab. 2002 May;282(5):E1139–46. doi:10.1152/ajpendo.00184.2001. PMID: 11934680.

Cappelletti M, Wallen K. Increasing women's sexual desire: the comparative effectiveness of estrogens and androgens. Horm Behav. 2016 Feb;78:178–93. doi:10.1016/j.yhbeh.2015.11.003. Epub 2015 Nov 14. PMID: 26589379; PMCID: PMC4720522.

Carr MC. The emergence of the metabolic syndrome with menopause. J Clin Endocrinol Metab. 2003 Jun;88(6):2404–11. doi:10.1210/jc.2003-030242. PMID: 12788835.

Chen C, Gong X, Yang X, Shang X, Du Q, Liao Q, Xie R, Chen Y, Xu J. The roles of estrogen and estrogen receptors in gastrointestinal disease. Oncol Lett. 2019 Dec;18(6):5673–80. doi:10.3892/ol.2019.10983. Epub 2019 Oct 11. PMID: 31788039; PMCID: PMC6865762.

Chidi-Ogbolu N, Baar K. Effect of estrogen on musculoskeletal performance and injury risk. Front Physiol. 2019 Jan 15;9:1834. doi:10.3389/fphys.2018.01834. PMID: 30697162; PMCID: PMC6341375.

Chlebowski RT, Cirillo DJ, Eaton CB, Stefanick ML, Pettinger M, Carbone LD, Johnson KC, Simon MS, Woods NF, Wactawski-Wende J. Estrogen alone and joint symptoms in the Women's Health Initiative randomized trial. Menopause. 2013 Jun;20(6):600–8. doi:10.1097/GME.0b013e31828392c4. PMID: 23511705; PMCID: PMC3855295.

Ciesielska A, Kusiak A, Ossowska A, Grzybowska ME. Changes in the oral cavity in menopausal women-a narrative review. Int J Environ Res Public Health. 2021 Dec 27;19(1):253. doi:10.3390/ijerph19010253. PMID: 35010513; PMCID: PMC8750983.

Cohen LS, Soares CN, Vitonis AF, Otto MW, Harlow BL. Risk for new onset of depression during the menopausal transition: the Harvard study of moods and cycles. Arch Gen Psychiatry. 2006 Apr;63(4):385–90. doi:10.1001/archpsyc.63.4.385. PMID: 16585467.

Coughlan GT, Betthauser TJ, Boyle R, et al. Association of age at menopause and hormone therapy use with tau and β-amyloid Positron Emission Tomography. JAMA Neurol. 2023;80(5):462–73. doi:10.1001/jamaneurol.2023.0455.

Cushman M, et al. Effect of postmenopausal hormones on inflammation-sensitive proteins: the Postmenopausal Estrogen/Progestin Interventions (PEPI) Study. Circulation. 1999;100(7):717–22.

d'Adesky ND, et al. Nicotine alters estrogen receptor-beta-regulated inflammasome activity and exacerbates ischemic brain damage in female rats. Int J Mol Sci. 2018;19(5):1330.

D'Alonzo M, Bounous VE, Villa M, Biglia N. Current evidence of the oncological benefit-risk profile of hormone replacement therapy. Medicina. 2019 Sep 7;55(9):573. doi:10.3390/medicina55090573. PMID: 31500261; PMCID: PMC6780494.

Da Silva AS, Baines G, Araklitis G, Robinson D, Cardozo L. Modern management of genitourinary syndrome of menopause. Fac Rev. 2021 Mar 3;10:25. doi:10.12703/r/10-25. PMID: 33718942; PMCID: PMC7946389.

De Paoli M, Zakharia A, Werstuck GH. The role of estrogen in insulin resistance: a review of clinical and preclinical data. Am J Pathol. 2021 Sep;191(9):1490–98. doi:10.1016/j.ajpath.2021.05.011. Epub 2021 Jun 5. PMID: 34102108.

Desai MK, Brinton RD. Autoimmune disease in women: endocrine transition and risk across the lifespan. Front Endocrinol. 2019 Apr 29;10:265. doi:10.3389/fendo.2019.00265. PMID: 31110493; PMCID: PMC6501433.

Edwards BJ, Li J. Endocrinology of menopause. Periodontol. 2013;61(1):177–94.

Farage MA, Miller KW, Maibach HI. Effects of menopause on autoimmune diseases. Expert Rev of Obst & Gyn. 2012;7(6):557–71. DOI:10.1586/eog.12.63.

Fiol G, Lete I, Nieto L, Santaballa A, Pla MJ, Baquedano L, Calaf J, Coronado P, de la Viuda E, Llaneza P, Otero B, Sánchez-Méndez S, Ramírez I, Mendoza N; HMT Eligibility Criteria Group. Associations between menopausal hormone therapy and colorectal, lung, or melanoma cancer recurrence and mortality: a narrative review. J Clin Med. 2023 Aug 12;12(16):5263. doi:10.3390/jcm12165263. PMID: 37629305; PMCID: PMC10455141.

Forbes AP. Fuller Albright. His concept of postmenopausal osteoporosis and what came of it. Clin Orthop Relat Res. 1991 Aug;269:128–41. PMID: 1864030.

Gaignard P, Liere P, Thérond P, Schumacher M, Slama A, Guennoun R. Role of sex hormones on brain mitochondrial function, with special reference to aging and neurodegenerative diseases. Front Aging Neurosci. 2017 Dec 7;9:406. doi:10.3389/fnagi.2017.00406. PMID: 29270123; PMCID: PMC5725410.

Gameiro CM, Romão F, Castelo-Branco C. Menopause and aging: changes in the immune system: a review. Maturitas. 2010 Dec;67(4):316–20. doi:10.1016/j.maturitas.2010.08.003. Epub 2010 Sep 1. PMID: 20813470.

Garcia-Segura LM, Diz-Chaves Y, Perez-Martin M, Darnaudéry M. Estradiol, insulin-like growth factor-I and brain aging. Psychoneuroendocrinology. 2007 Aug;32 Suppl 1:S57–61. doi:10.1016/j.psyneuen.2007.03.001. Epub 2007 Jul 6. PMID: 17618061.

Georgiadou P, Sbarouni E. Effect of hormone replacement therapy on inflammatory biomarkers. Adv Clin Chem. 2009;47:59–93. doi:10.1016/s0065-2423(09)47003-3. PMID: 19634777.

Giannoni E, et al. Estradiol and progesterone strongly inhibit the innate immune response of mononuclear cells in newborns. Infect Immun. 2011;79(7):2690–98.

Giefing-Kröll C, Berger P, Lepperdinger G, Grubeck-Loebenstein B. How sex and age affect immune responses, susceptibility to infections, and response to vaccination. Aging Cell. 2015;14:309–21. https://doi.org/10.1111/acel.12326.

Giordano S, Hage FG, Xing D, Chen YF, Allon S, Chen C, Oparil S. Estrogen and cardiovascular disease: is timing everything? Am J Med Sci. 2015 Jul;350(1):27–35. doi:10.1097/MAJ.0000000000000512. PMID: 26110752; PMCID: PMC4490077.

Girard R, Météreau E, Thomas J, Pugeat M, Qu C, Dreher JC. Hormone therapy at early post-menopause increases cognitive control-related prefrontal activity. Sci Rep. 2017 Mar 21;7:44917. doi:10.1038/srep44917. PMID: 28322310; PMCID: PMC5359606.

Gordon JL, Rubinow DR, Eisenlohr-Moul TA, Xia K, Schmidt PJ, Girdler SS. Efficacy of transdermal estradiol and micronized progesterone in the prevention of depressive symptoms in the menopause transition: a randomized clinical trial. JAMA Psychiatry. 2018 Feb 1;75(2):149–57. doi:10.1001/jamapsychiatry.2017.3998. PMID: 29322164; PMCID: PMC5838629.

Grymowicz M, Rudnicka E, Podfigurna A, Napierala P, Smolarczyk R, Smolarczyk K, Meczekalski B. Hormonal effects on hair follicles. Int J Mol Sci. 2020 Jul 28;21(15):5342. doi:10.3390/ijms21155342. PMID: 32731328; PMCID: PMC7432488.

Hodis HN, Mack WJ. Menopausal hormone replacement therapy and reduction of all-cause mortality and cardiovascular disease: it is about time and timing. Cancer J. 2022 May–Jun 01;28(3):208–23. doi:10.1097/PPO.0000000000000591. PMID: 35594469; PMCID: PMC9178928.

Hormone therapy appears to reduce risk of shoulder pain in older women. Duke Health. October 11, 2022. https://corporate.dukehealth.org/news/hormone-therapy-appears-reduce-risk-shoulder-pain-older-women.

Iorga A, Cunningham CM, Moazeni S, Ruffenach G, Umar S, Eghbali M. The protective role of estrogen and estrogen receptors in cardiovascular disease and the controversial use of estrogen therapy. Biol Sex Differ. 2017 Oct 24;8(1):33. doi:10.1186/s13293-017-0152-8. PMID: 29065927; PMCID: PMC5655818.

Iyer TK, Thacker HL. Menopause. In: Falcone T, Hurd WW. Clinical reproductive medicine and surgery. Cham: Springer, 2022. https://doi.org/10.1007/978-3-030-99596-6_9.

Jacenik D, Zielińska M, Mokrowiecka A, et al. G protein-coupled estrogen receptor mediates anti-inflammatory action in Crohn's disease. Sci Rep. 2019;9:6749. https://doi.org/10.1038/s41598-019-43233-3.

Javed AA, Mayhew AJ, Shea AK, Raina P. Association between hormone therapy and muscle mass in postmenopausal women: a systematic review and meta-analysis. JAMA Netw Open. 2019 Aug 2;2(8):e1910154. doi:10.1001/jamanetworkopen.2019.10154. PMID: 31461147; PMCID: PMC6716293.

Jiang L, Fei H, Tong J, Zhou J, Zhu J, Jin X, Shi Z, Zhou Y, Ma X, Yu H, Yang J, Zhang S. Hormone replacement therapy reverses gut microbiome and serum metabolome alterations in premature ovarian insufficiency. Front Endocrinol. 2021 Dec 23;12:794496. doi:10.3389/fendo.2021.794496. PMID: 35002971; PMCID: PMC8733385.

Kim SH, Kang BM, Chae HD, Kim CH. The association between serum estradiol level and hearing sensitivity in postmenopausal women. Obstet Gynecol. 2002 May;99(5 Pt 1):726–30. doi:10.1016/s0029-7844(02)01963-4. PMID: 11978279.

Lamkanfi M, Dixit VM. Mechanisms and functions of inflammasomes. Cell. 2014;157(5):1013–22.

Leite G, Barlow GM, Parodi G, Pimentel ML, Chang C, Hosseini A, Wang J, Pimentel M, Mathur R. Duodenal microbiome changes in postmenopausal women: effects of hormone therapy and implications for cardiovascular risk. Menopause. 2022 Jan 24;29(3):264–75. doi:10.1097/GME.0000000000001917. PMID: 35213514; PMCID: PMC8862775.

Lejri I, Grimm A, Eckert A. Mitochondria, estrogen and female brain aging. Front Aging Neurosci. 2018 Apr 27;10:124. doi:10.3389/fnagi.2018.00124. PMID: 29755342; PMCID: PMC5934418.

Li F, Boon ACM, Michelson AP, et al. Estrogen hormone is an essential sex factor inhibiting inflammation and immune response in COVID-19. Sci Rep. 2022;12:9462. https://doi.org/10.1038/s41598-022-13585-4.

Li G, Yin J, Gao J, Cheng TS, Pavlos NJ, Zhang C, Zheng MH. Subchondral bone in osteoarthritis: insight into risk factors and microstructural changes. Arthritis Res Ther. 2013;15(6):223. doi:10.1186/ar4405. PMID: 24321104; PMCID: PMC4061721.

Looijer-van Langen M, Hotte N, Dieleman LA, Albert E, Mulder C, Madsen KL. Estrogen receptor-β signaling modulates epithelial barrier function. Am J Physiol Gastrointest Liver Physiol. 2011 Apr;300(4):G621–6. doi:10.1152/ajpgi.00274.2010. Epub 2011 Jan 20. PMID: 21252046.

Manyonda I, Sinai Talaulikar V, Pirhadi R, Ward J, Banerjee D, Onwude J. Could perimenopausal estrogen prevent breast cancer? exploring the differential effects of estrogen-only versus combined hormone replacement therapy. J Clin Med Res. 2022 Jan;14(1):1–7. doi:10.14740/jocmr4646. Epub 2022 Jan 29. PMID: 35211211; PMCID: PMC8827222.

Mauvais-Jarvis F, Clegg DJ, Hevener AL. The role of estrogens in control of energy balance and glucose homeostasis. Endocr Rev. 2013 Jun;34(3):309–38. doi:10.1210/er.2012-1055. Epub 2013 Mar 4. PMID: 23460719; PMCID: PMC3660717.

Mikkola TS, Savolainen-Peltonen H, Tuomikoski P, Hoti F, Vattulainen P, Gissler M, Ylikorkala O. Reduced risk of breast cancer mortality in women using postmenopausal hormone therapy: a Finnish nationwide comparative study. Menopause. 2016 Nov;23(11):1199–1203. doi:10.1097/GME.0000000000000698. PMID: 27465718.

Miller AP, Chen YF, Xing D, Feng W, Oparil S. Hormone replacement therapy and inflammation: interactions i n cardiovascular disease. Hypertension. 2003 Oct;42(4):657–63. doi:10.1161/01.HYP.0000085560.02979.0C. Epub 2003 Aug 11. PMID: 12913055.

Miller S. Listening to estrogen hormones have always been a third rail in female mental health. New York. December 21, 2018. https://www.thecut.com/2018/12/is-estrogen-the-key-to-understanding-womens-mental-health.html.

Miller S. Women battling their hormones are demanding to be heard. New York. January 10, 2019. https://www.thecut.com/2019/01/estrogen-and-mental-health-women-share-their-stories.html.

Mooga, Ved P, et al. Estrogen and mitochondrial function in disease. Mitoch Dis, InTech. Aug. 2018. Crossref, doi:10.5772/intechopen.73015.

Mosconi L, Berti V, Guyara-Quinn C, McHugh P, Petrongolo G, Osorio RS, et al. Perimenopause and emergence of an Alzheimer's bioenergetic phenotype in brain and periphery. PLoS One. 2018;12:e0185926. 10.1371/journal.pone.0185926

Nuzzi R, Caselgrandi P. Sex hormones and their effects on ocular disorders and pathophysiology: current aspects and our experience. Intl J Molec Sci. 2022;23(6):3269. https://doi.org/10.3390/ijms23063269.

Overview of osteoporosis. https://www.niams.nih.gov/health-topics/osteoporosis#:~:text=Osteoporosis%20is%20a%20bone%20disease,of%20fractures%20(broken%20bones).

Pfeilschifter J, Köditz R, Pfohl M, Schatz H. Changes in pro-inflammatory cytokine activity after menopause. Endocr Rev. 2002 Feb;23(1):90–119. doi:10.1210/edrv.23.1.0456. PMID: 11844745.

Phillips SM, Sherwin BB. Effects of estrogen on memory function in surgically menopausal women. Psychoneuro-endocrinology. 1992 Oct;17(5):485–95. doi:10.1016/0306-4530(92)90007-t. PMID: 1484915.

Primary ovarian insufficiency. Mayo Foundation for Medical Education and Research. 2021 [cited 2023 Jun 9]. https://www.mayoclinic.org/diseases-conditions/premature-ovarian-failure/symptoms-causes/syc-20354683.

Robinson D, Toozs-Hobson P, Cardozo L. The effect of hormones on the lower urinary tract. Meno Intl: The Integr J Postreprod Health. 2013;19(4):155–62. doi:10.1177/1754045313511398

Rzepecki AK, Murase JE, Juran R, Fabi SG, McLellan BN. Estrogen-deficient skin: the role of topical therapy. Int J Women's Dermatol. 2019 Mar 15;5(2):85–90. doi:10.1016/j.ijwd.2019.01.001. PMID: 30997378; PMCID: PMC6451761.

Sammaritano LR. Menopause in patients with autoimmune diseases. Autoimmun Rev. 2012 May;11(6–7):A430–36. doi:10.1016/j.autrev.2011.11.006. Epub 2011 Nov 18. PMID: 22120060.

Sarrel PM. Effects of hormone replacement therapy on sexual psychophysiology and behavior in postmenopause. J Women's Health Gend Based Med. 2000;9(Suppl 1):S25–32. doi:10.1089/152460900318830. Erratum in: J Women's Health Gend Based Med. 2001 Jan-Feb;10(1):91. PMID: 10695871.

Schmidl D, Szalai L, Kiss OG, Schmetterer L, Garhöfer G. A phase II, multicenter, randomized, placebo-controlled, double-masked trial of a topical estradiol ophthalmic formulation in postmenopausal women with moderate-to-severe dry eye disease. Adv Ther. 2021 Apr;38(4):1975–86. doi:10.1007/s12325-021-01680-3. Epub 2021 Mar 12. PMID: 33710587.

Seifert-Klauss V, Prior JC. Progesterone and bone: actions promoting bone health in women. J Osteoporos. 2010 Oct 31;2010:845180. doi:10.4061/2010/845180. PMID: 21052538; PMCID: PMC2968416.

Sharma A, Davies R, Kapoor A, Islam H, Webber L, Jayasena CN. The effect of hormone replacement therapy on cognition and mood. Clin Endocrinol. 2023;98:285–95. doi:10.1111/cen.14856.

Singh V, Park YJ, Lee G, Unno T, Shin JH. Dietary regulations for microbiota dysbiosis among post-menopausal women with type 2 diabetes. Crit Rev Food Sci Nutr. 2022 May 30:1–16. doi:10.1080/10408398.2022.2076651. Epub ahead of print. PMID: 35635755.

Sites CK, Toth MJ, Cushman M, L'Hommedieu GD, Tchernof A, Tracy RP, Poehlman ET. Menopause-related differences in inflammation markers and their relationship to body fat distribution and insulin-stimulated glucose disposal. Fertil Steril. 2002 Jan;77(1):128–35. doi:10.1016/s0015-0282(01)02934-x. PMID: 11779602.

Ślebioda Z, Szponar E. Burning mouth syndrome: a common dental problem in perimenopausal women. Prz Menopauzalny. 2014 Jun;13(3):198–202. doi:10.5114/pm.2014.43825. Epub 2014 Jun 30. PMID: 26327855; PMCID: PMC4520363.

Smith A, Contreras C, Ko KH, Chow J, Dong X, Tuo B, Zhang HH, Chen DB, Dong H. Gender-specific protection of estrogen against gastric acid-induced duodenal injury: stimulation of duodenal mucosal bicarbonate secretion. Endocrinology. 2008 Sep;149(9):4554–66. doi:10.1210/en.2007-1597. Epub 2008 May 22. PMID: 18499763; PMCID: PMC2553385.

Sniekers YH, Weinans H, van Osch GJ, van Leeuwen JP. Oestrogen is important for maintenance of cartilage and subchondral bone in a murine model of knee osteoarthritis. Arthritis Res Ther. 2010;12(5):R182. doi:10.1186/ar3148. Epub 2010 Oct 5. PMID: 20923566; PMCID: PMC2991014.

Stubbins RE, Holcomb VB, Hong J, Núñez NP. Estrogen modulates abdominal adiposity and protects female mice from obesity and impaired glucose tolerance. Eur J Nutr. 2012 Oct;51(7):861–70. doi:10.1007/s00394-011-0266-4. Epub 2011 Nov 1. PMID: 22042005.

Tiidus PM. Benefits of estrogen replacement for skeletal muscle mass and function in post-menopausal females: evidence from human and animal studies. Eurasian J Med. 2011 Aug;43(2):109–14. doi:10.5152/eajm.2011.24. PMID: 25610174; PMCID: PMC4261347.

Vajaranant TS, Pasquale LR. Estrogen deficiency accelerates aging of the optic nerve. Menopause: J N Am Meno Soc. 2012 Aug;19(8):942–47. DOI:10.1097/gme.0b013e3182443137.

Vegeto E, Benedusi V, Maggi A. Estrogen anti-inflammatory activity in brain: a therapeutic opportunity for menopause and neurodegenerative diseases. Front Neuroendocrinol. 2008;29(4):507–19.

Visser M, Langlois J, Guralnik JM, Cauley JA, Kronmal RA, Robbins J, Williamson JD, Harris TB. High body fatness, but not low fat-free mass, predicts disability in older men and women: the Cardiovascular Health Study. Am J Clin Nutr. 1998 Sep;68(3):584–90. doi:10.1093/ajcn/68.3.584. PMID: 9734734.

Wei Yu, et al. Estrogen prevents cellular senescence and bone loss through Usp10-dependent p53 degradation in osteocytes and osteoblasts: the role of estrogen in bone cell senescence. Cell and Tiss Res. 2021 Nov;386(2):297+.

Yes, you can have better sex in midlife and in the years beyond. Harvard Health. September 30, 2021. https://www.health.harvard.edu/womens-health/yes-you-can-have-better-sex-in-midlie-and-in-the-years-beyond.

Zárate S, Astiz M, Magnani N, Imsen M, Merino F, Álvarez S, Reinés A, Seilicovich A. Hormone deprivation alters mitochondrial function and lipid profile in the hippocampus. J Endocrinol. 2017 Apr;233(1):1–14. doi:10.1530/JOE-16-0451. Epub 2017 Jan 27. PMID: 28130408.

Zhipeng T, Zhiyong C. Hormonal regulation of metabolism—recent lessons learned from insulin and estrogen. Clin Sci. 2023 March;137(6):415–34. doi:https://doi.org/10.1042/CS20210519

PART II: HEALTHY AGING THROUGH MIDLIFE AND MENOPAUSE: OPTIMAL METABOLIC HEALTH VIA NUTRITION, GUT, LIFESTYLE, ADRENALS, AND THYROID STATUS

Chapter Five: The Importance of Metabolic Health

Baylis D, Bartlett DB, Patel HP, Roberts HC. Understanding how we age: insights into inflammaging. Longev Healthspan. 2013 May 2;2(1):8. doi:10.1186/2046-2395-2-8. PMID: 24472098; PMCID: PMC3922951.

Bermingham KM, Linenberg I, Hall WL, Kadé K, Franks PW, Davies R, Wolf J, Hadjigeorgiou G, Asnicar F, Segata N, Manson JE, Newson LR, Delahanty LM, Ordovas JM, Chan AT, Spector TD, Valdes AM, Berry SE. Menopause is associated with postprandial metabolism, metabolic health and lifestyle: The ZOE PREDICT study. EBioMedicine. 2022 Nov;85:104303. doi:10.1016/j.ebiom.2022.104303. Epub 2022 Oct 18. PMID: 36270905; PMCID: PMC9669773.

de Zoete MR, Palm NW, Zhu S, Flavell RA. Inflammasomes. Cold Spring Harb Perspect Biol. 2014 Oct 16;6(12):a016287. doi:10.1101/cshperspect.a016287. PMID: 25324215; PMCID: PMC4292152.

Ferrucci L, Fabbri E. Inflammageing: chronic inflammation in ageing, cardiovascular disease, and frailty. Nat Rev Cardiol. 2018 Sep;15(9):505–22. doi:10.1038/s41569-018-0064-2. PMID: 30065258; PMCID: PMC6146930.

Franceschi C, Garagnani P, Parini P, Giuliani C, Santoro A. Inflammaging: a new immune-metabolic viewpoint for age-related diseases. Nat Rev Endocrinol. 2018 Oct;14(10):576–90. doi:10.1038/s41574-018-0059-4. PMID: 30046148.

McCarthy M, Raval AP. The peri-menopause in a woman's life: a systemic inflammatory phase that enables later neurodegenerative disease. J Neuroinflammation. 2020 Oct 23;17(1):317. doi:10.1186/s12974-020-01998-9. PMID: 33097048; PMCID: PMC7585188.

Chapter Six: Curating Nutrition for Midlife

A metabolomics comparison of plant-based meat and grass-fed meat indicates large nutritional differences despite comparable Nutrition Facts panels. https://www.nature.com/articles/s41598-021-93100-3.

Alves BC, Silva TR, Spritzer PM. Sedentary lifestyle and high-carbohydrate intake are associated with low-grade chronic inflammation in post-menopause: a cross-sectional study. Rev Bras Ginecol Obstet. 2016 Jul;38(7):317–24. doi:10.1055/s-0036-1584582. Epub 2016 Jul 15. PMID: 27420776.

Astrup A, Magkos F, Bier D, et al. Saturated fats and health: a reassessment and proposal for food-based recommendations. J Am Coll Cardiol. 2020 Aug;76(7):844–57. https://doi.org/10.1016/j.jacc.2020.05.077.

Blom WA, Lluch A, Stafleu A, Vinoy S, Holst JJ, Schaafsma G, Hendriks HF. Effect of a high-protein breakfast on the postprandial ghrelin response. Am J Clin Nutr. 2006 Feb;83(2):211–20. doi:10.1093/ajcn/83.2.211. PMID: 16469977.

Devries MC, et al. Changes in kidney function do not differ between healthy adults consuming higher- compared with lower- or normal-protein diets: a systematic review and meta-analysis. J Nutr. 2018 Nov 1;148(11):1760–75. DOI:10.1093/jn/nxy197.

Dougkas A, Östman E. Protein-enriched liquid preloads varying in macronutrient content modulate appetite and appetite-regulating hormones in healthy adults. J Nutr.

2016 Mar;146(3):637–45. doi:10.3945/jn.115.217224. Epub 2016 Jan 20. PMID: 26791555.

Elsworth RL, Monge A, Perry R, Hinton EC, Flynn AN, Whitmarsh A, Hamilton-Shield JP, Lawrence NS, Brunstrom JM. The effect of intermittent fasting on appetite: a systematic review and meta-analysis. Nutrients. 2023;15:2604. https://doi.org/10.3390/nu15112604.

Ford C, Chang S, Vitolins MZ, Fenton JI, Howard BV, Rhee JJ, Stefanick M, Chen B, Snetselaar L, Urrutia R, Frazier-Wood AC. Consuming a reduced-carbohydrate diet, with moderate fat and high protein intake, may decrease the risk of weight gain in post-menopausal women: evaluation of diet pattern and weight gain in postmenopausal women enrolled in the Women's Health Initiative Observational Study. Br J Nutr. 2017 Apr;117(8):1189–97. doi:10.1017/S0007114517000952. Epub 2017 May 16. PMID: 28509665; PMCID: PMC5728369.

Fromentin C, Tomé D, Nau F, Flet L, Luengo C, Azzout-Marniche D, Sanders P, Fromentin G, Gaudichon C. Dietary proteins contribute little to glucose production, even under optimal gluconeogenic conditions in healthy humans. Diabetes. 2013 May;62(5):1435–42. doi:10.2337/db12-1208. Epub 2012 Dec 28. PMID: 23274906; PMCID: PMC3636601.

Hruby A, Sahni S, Bolster D, Jacques PF. Protein intake and functional integrity in aging: the Framingham Heart Study offspring. J Geront: Series A. 2020 Jan;75(1):123–30. https://doi.org/10.1093/gerona/gly201.

Johnston BC, Zeraatkar D, Han MA, Vernooij RWM, Valli C, El Dib R, Marshall C, Stover PJ, Fairweather-Taitt S, Wójcik G, Bhatia F, de Souza R, Brotons C, Meerpohl JJ, Patel CJ, Djulbegovic B, Alonso-Coello P, Bala MM, Guyatt GH. Unprocessed red meat and processed meat consumption: dietary guideline recommendations from the Nutritional Recommendations (NutriRECS) Consortium. Ann Intern Med. 2019 Nov 19;171(10):756–64. doi:10.7326/M19-1621. Epub 2019 Oct 1. PMID: 31569235.

Lejeune MP, Westerterp KR, Adam TC, Luscombe-Marsh ND, Westerterp-Plantenga MS. Ghrelin and glucagon-like peptide 1 concentrations, 24-h satiety, and energy and substrate metabolism during a high-protein diet and measured in a respiration chamber. Am J Clin Nutr. 2006 Jan;83(1):89–94. doi:10.1093/ajcn/83.1.89. PMID: 16400055.

Ma Y, Sun L, Mu Z. Effects of different weight loss dietary interventions on body mass index and glucose and lipid metabolism in obese patients. Medicine. 2023 Mar;102(13):pe33254. DOI:10.1097/MD.0000000000033254.

Perna S, Avanzato I, Nichetti M, D'Antona G, Negro M, Rondanelli M. Association between dietary patterns of meat and fish consumption with bone mineral density or fracture risk: a systematic literature. Nutrients. 2017 Sep 18;9(9):1029. doi:10.3390/nu9091029. PMID: 29358568; PMCID: PMC5622789.

Pesta DH, Samuel VT. A high-protein diet for reducing body fat: mechanisms and possible caveats. Nutr Metab. 2014 Nov 19;11(1):53. doi:10.1186/1743-7075-11-53. PMID: 25489333; PMCID: PMC4258944.

Rodgers D, Wolf R. Sacred Cow. Dallas: BenBella, 2021.

Rogeri PS, Zanella R Jr, Martins GL, Garcia MDA, Leite G, Lugaresi R, Gasparini SO, Sperandio GA, Ferreira LHB, Souza-Junior TP, Lancha AH Jr. Strategies to prevent sarcopenia in the aging process: role of protein intake and exercise. Nutrients. 2021 Dec 23;14(1):52. doi:10.3390/nu14010052. PMID: 35010928; PMCID: PMC8746908.

Scott T. Collagen and gelatin lower serotonin: does this increase your anxiety and depression? Anxiety Nutrition Solutions. September 29, 2017. https://www.everywomanover29.com/blog/collagen-gelatin-lower-serotonin-increase-anxiety-depression.

Walton C, Godsland IF, Proudler AJ, Wynn V, Stevenson JC. The effects of the menopause on insulin sensitivity, secretion and elimination in non-obese, healthy women. Euro J Clin Inv. 1993;23:466–73.

Weigle DS, Breen PA, Matthys CC, Callahan HS, Meeuws KE, Burden VR, Purnell JQ. A high-protein diet induces sustained reductions in appetite, ad libitum caloric intake, and body weight despite compensatory changes in diurnal plasma leptin and ghrelin concentrations. Am J Clin Nutr. 2005 Jul;82(1):41–48. doi:10.1093/ajcn.82.1.41. PMID: 16002798.

What the food industry does not want you to know about climate change, with Dr. Frank Mitloehner. The Dr. Gabrielle Lyon Show. October 2022. https://open.spotify.com/episode/0knczKa9COhyHQTI6B-D2CS?si=63818a7350454de1

Chapter Seven: The Microbiome in Midlife: Why Daily Poops Are Essential

Arlinghaus KR, Johnston CA. The importance of creating habits and routine. Am J Lifestyle Med. 2018 Dec 29;13(2):142–44. doi:10.1177/1559827618818044. PMID: 30800018; PMCID: PMC6378489.

Asanuma K, Iijima K, Shimosegawa T. Gender difference in gastro-esophageal reflux diseases. World J Gastroenterol. 2016 Feb 7;22(5):1800–10. doi:10.3748/wjg.v22.i5.1800. PMID: 26855539; PMCID: PMC4724611.

Ashraf MS, Vongpatanasin W. Estrogen and hypertension. Curr Hypertens Rep. 2006 Oct;8(5):368–76. doi:10.1007/s11906-006-0080-1. PMID: 16965722.

Baker JM, Al-Nakkash L, Herbst-Kralovetz MM. Estrogen-gut microbiome axis: physiological and clinical implications. Maturitas. 2017 Sep;103:45–53. doi:10.1016/j.maturitas.2017.06.025. Epub 2017 Jun 23. PMID: 28778332.

Beta 3 adrenergic receptor stimulating agent. https://www.sciencedirect.com/topics/medicine-and-dentistry/beta-3-adrenergic-receptor-stimulating-agent.

Boland M. Human digestion: a processing perspective. J Sci Food Agric. 2016 May;96(7):2275–83. doi:10.1002/jsfa.7601. Epub 2016 Feb 5. PMID: 26711173.

Browning KN, Travagli RA. Central nervous system control of gastrointestinal motility and secretion and modulation of gastrointestinal functions. Compr Physiol. 2014 Oct;4(4):1339–68. doi:10.1002/cphy.c130055. PMID: 25428846; PMCID: PMC4858318.

Chen C, et al. The roles of estrogen and estrogen receptors in gastrointestinal disease. Oncol Lett. 2019;18(6):5673–80.

Cherpak CE. Mindful eating: a review of how the stress-digestion-mindfulness triad may modulate and improve gastrointestinal and digestive function. Integr Med. 2019 Aug;18(4):48–53. PMID: 32549835; PMCID: PMC7219460.

Cody JD, Jacobs ML, Richardson K, Moehrer B, Hextall A. Oestrogen therapy for urinary incontinence in postmenopausal women. Cochrane Database Syst Rev. 2012 Oct 17;10(10):CD001405. doi:10.1002/14651858.CD001405.pub3. PMID: 23076892; PMCID: PMC7086391.

Dashnyam P, Mudududdla R, Hsieh TJ, et al. β-Glucuronidases of opportunistic bacteria are the major contributors to xenobiotic-induced toxicity in the gut. Sci Rep. 2018;8:16372. https://doi.org/10.1038/s41598-018-34678-z.

Dave M, Higgins PD, Middha S, Rioux KP. The human gut microbiome: current knowledge, challenges, and future directions. Transl Res. 2012 Oct;160(4):246–57. doi:10.1016/j.trsl.2012.05.003. Epub 2012 Jun 7. PMID: 22683238.

de Vos WM, Tilg H, Van Hul M, Cani PD. Gut microbiome and health: mechanistic insights. Gut. 2022 May;71(5):1020–32. doi:10.1136/gutjnl-2021-326789. Epub 2022 Feb 1. PMID: 35105664; PMCID: PMC8995832.

Definition & facts for constipation. https://www.niddk.nih.gov/health-information/digestive-diseases/constipation/definition-facts

Gao R, Tao Y, Zhou C, Li J, Wang X, Chen L, Li F, Guo L. Exercise therapy in patients with constipation: a systematic review and meta-analysis of randomized controlled trials. Scand J Gastroenterol. 2019 Feb;54(2):169–77. doi:10.1080/00365521.2019.1568544. Epub 2019 Mar 7. PMID: 30843436.

Gordon JL, Girdler SS. Hormone replacement therapy in the treatment of perimenopausal depression. Curr Psychiatry Rep. 2014 Dec;16(12):517. doi:10.1007/s11920-014-0517-1. PMID: 25308388.

Heitkemper MM, Chang L. Do fluctuations in ovarian hormones affect gastrointestinal symptoms in women with irritable bowel syndrome? Gend Med. 2009;6 Suppl 2(Suppl 2):152–67. doi:10.1016/j.genm.2009.03.004. PMID: 19406367; PMCID: PMC3322543.

Hendrix SL, Cochrane BB, Nygaard IE, et al. Effects of estrogen with and without progestin on urinary incontinence. JAMA. 2005;293(8):935–48. doi:10.1001/jama.293.8.935.

Hermann M, Flammer A, Lüscher TF. Nitric oxide in hypertension. J Clin Hypertens. 2006 Dec;8 (12 Suppl 4):17–29. doi:10.1111/j.1524-6175.2006.06032.x. PMID: 17170603; PMCID: PMC8109558.

Hodges RE, Minich DM. Modulation of metabolic detoxification pathways using foods and food-derived components: a scientific review with clinical application. J Nutr Metab. 2015;2015:760689. doi:10.1155/2015/760689. Epub 2015 Jun 16. PMID: 26167297; PMCID: PMC4488002.

Jebb SA, Moore MS. Contribution of a sedentary lifestyle and inactivity to the etiology of overweight and obesity: current evidence and research issues. Med Sci Sports Exerc. 1999 Nov;31(11 Suppl):S534–41. doi:10.1097/00005768-199911001-00008. PMID: 10593524.

Katschinski M. Nutritional implications of cephalic phase gastrointestinal responses. Appetite. 2000 Apr;34(2):189–96. doi:10.1006/appe.1999.0280. PMID: 10744909.

Koutoukidis DA, Jebb SA, Zimmerman M, Otunla A, Henry JA, Ferrey A, Schofield E, Kinton J, Aveyard P, Marchesi JR. The association of weight loss with changes in the gut microbiota diversity, composition, and intestinal permeability: a systematic review and meta-analysis. Gut Microbes. 2022 Jan-Dec;14(1):2020068. doi:10.1080/19490976.2021.2020068. PMID: 35040746; PMCID: PMC8796717.

Lewis G, Wang B, Shafiei Jahani P, Hurrell BP, Banie H, Aleman Muench GR, Maazi H, Helou DG, Howard E, Galle-Treger L, Lo R, Santosh S, Baltus A, Bongers G, San-Mateo L, Gilliland FD, Rehan VK, Soroosh P, Akbari O. Dietary fiber-induced microbial short chain fatty acids suppress ILC2-dependent airway inflammation. Front Immunol. 2019 Sep;18(10):2051. doi:10.3389/fimmu.2019.02051. PMID: 31620118; PMCID: PMC6760365.

Magnon V, Dutheil F, Vallet GT. Benefits from one session of deep and slow breathing on vagal tone and anxiety in young and older adults. Sci Rep. 2021 Sep 29;11(1):19267. doi:10.1038/s41598-021-98736-9. PMID: 34588511; PMCID: PMC8481564.

Margolis KG, Cryan JF, Mayer EA. The microbiota-gut-brain axis: from motility to mood. Gastroenterology. 2021 Apr;160(5):1486–1501. doi:10.1053/j.gastro.2020.10.066. Epub 2021 Jan 22. PMID: 33493503; PMCID: PMC8634751.

Maruti SS, Li L, Chang JL, Prunty J, Schwarz Y, Li SS, King IB, Potter JD, Lampe JW. Dietary and demographic correlates of serum beta-glucuronidase activity. Nutr Cancer. 2010;62(2):208–19. doi:10.1080/01635580903305375. PMID: 20099195; PMCID: PMC2858007

Maynard C, Weinkove D. The gut microbiota and ageing. Subcell Biochem. 2018;90:351–71. doi:10.1007/978-981-13-2835-0_12. PMID: 30779015.

McCully KS, Jackson S. Hormone replacement therapy and the bladder. J Br Menopause Soc. 2004 Mar;10(1):30–2. doi:10.1258/136218004322986753. PMID: 15107209.

Mörkl S, Butler MI, Lackner S. Advances in the gut microbiome and mood disorders. Curr Opin Psychiatry. 2023 Jan 1;36(1):1–7. doi:10.1097/YCO.0000000000000829. PMID: 36131643.

Neuman H, Debelius JW, Knight R, Koren O. Microbial endocrinology: the interplay between the microbiota and the endocrine system. FEMS Microbiol Rev. 2015 Jul;39(4):509–21. doi:10.1093/femsre/fuu010. Epub 2015 Feb 19. PMID: 25701044.

Nie X, et al. Effects of estrogen on the gastrointestinal tract. Dig Dis Sci. 2018;63:583–96.

Park JH, Hong JY, Han K, Han SW, Chun EM. Relationship between hormone replacement therapy and spinal osteoarthritis: a nationwide health survey analysis of the elderly Korean population. BMJ Open. 2017 Nov 9;7(11):e018063. doi:10.1136/bmjopen-2017-018063. PMID: 29127229; PMCID: PMC5695470.

Peters BA, Santoro N, Kaplan RC, Qi Q. Spotlight on the gut microbiome in menopause: current insights. Int J Women's Health. 2022 Aug;14:1059–72. doi:10.2147/IJWH.S340491. PMID: 35983178; PMCID: PMC9379122.

Reynoso-Garcia J, et al. A complete guide to human microbiomes: body niches, transmission, development, dysbiosis, and restoration. Front Syst Biol. 2022 Jul;2. https://www.frontiersin.org/articles/10.3389/fsysb.2022.951403/full

Rollet M, Bohn T, Vahid F, on Behalf of the Oriscav Working Group. Association between dietary factors and constipation in adults living in Luxembourg and taking part in the ORISCAV-LUX 2 survey. Nutrients. 2021 Dec 28;14(1):122. doi:10.3390/nu14010122. PMID: 35010999; PMCID: PMC8746799.

Roman-Blas JA, Castañeda S, Largo R, Herrero-Beaumont G. Osteoarthritis associated with estrogen deficiency. Arthritis Res Ther. 2009;11(5):241. doi:10.1186/ar2791. Epub 2009 Sep 21. PMID: 19804619; PMCID: PMC2787275.

Strandwitz P. Neurotransmitter modulation by the gut microbiota. Brain Res. 2018 Aug 15;1693(Pt B):128–133. doi:10.1016/j.brainres.2018.03.015. PMID: 29903615; PMCID: PMC6005194.

Thomas-White K, Taege S, Limeira R, Brincat C, Joyce C, Hilt EE, MacDaniel L, Radek KA, Brubaker L, Mueller ER, Wolfe AJ. Vaginal estrogen therapy is associated with increased Lactobacillus in the urine of postmenopausal women with overactive bladder symptoms. Am J Obstet Gynecol. 2020 Nov;223(5):727.e1-727.e11. doi:10.1016/j.ajog.2020.08.006. Epub 2020 Aug 11. PMID: 32791124; PMCID: PMC7609597.

Turnbaugh PJ, Ley RE, Hamady M, Fraser-Liggett CM, Knight R, Gordon JI. The human microbiome project. Nature. 2007 Oct 18;449(7164):804–10. doi:10.1038/nature06244. PMID: 17943116; PMCID: PMC3709439.

Vandeputte D, Falony G, Vieira-Silva S, Tito RY, Joossens M, Raes J. Stool consistency is strongly associated with gut microbiota richness and composition, enterotypes and bacterial growth rates. Gut. 2016 Jan;65(1):57–62. doi:10.1136/gutjnl-2015-309618. Epub 2015 Jun 11. PMID: 26069274; PMCID: PMC4717365.

Yang J, Wang HP, Zhou L, Xu CF. Effect of dietary fiber on constipation: a meta-analysis. World J Gastroenterol. 2012 Dec 28;18(48):7378–83. doi:10.3748/wjg.v18.i48.7378. PMID: 23326148; PMCID: PMC3544045.

Yaoita F, Watanabe K, Kimura I, Miyazawa M, Tsuchiya S, Kanzaki M, Tsuchiya M, Tan-No K. Impact of habitual chewing on gut motility via microbiota transition. Sci Rep. 2022 Aug 15;12(1):13819. doi:10.1038/s41598-022-18095-x. PMID: 35970869; PMCID: PMC9378666.

Chapter Eight: Lifestyle Foundations in Midlife: Adapting the Pillars of Sleep, Stress Management, Movement, Community, and Mind-Set

Alvord VM, Kantra EJ, Pendergast JS. Estrogens and the circadian system. Semin Cell Dev Biol. 2022 Jun;126:56–65. doi:10.1016/j.semcdb.2021.04.010. Epub 2021 May 9. PMID: 33975754; PMCID: PMC8573061.

Baker A, Simpson S, Dawson D. Sleep disruption and mood changes associated with menopause. J Psychosom Res. 1997 Oct;43(4):359–69. doi:10.1016/s0022-3999(97)00126-8. PMID: 9330235.

Burke L. The rise of midlife social anxiety—and how to stop scrolling. The Telegraph. August 2, 2022. https://www.telegraph.co.uk/health-fitness/body/rise-midlife-social-media-anxiety-how-stop-scrolling.

Burrup R, Tucker LA, LE Cheminant JD, Bailey BW. Strength training and body composition in middle-age women. J Sports Med Phys Fitness. 2018 Jan–Feb;58(1-2):82–91. doi:10.23736/S0022-4707.17.06706-8. Epub 2017 Feb 8. PMID: 28181774.

Caufriez A, Leproult R, L'Hermite-Balériaux M, Kerkhofs M, Copinschi G. Progesterone prevents sleep disturbances and modulates GH, TSH, and melatonin secretion in postmenopausal women. J Clin Endocrinol Metab. 2011 Apr;96(4):E614–23. doi:10.1210/jc.2010-2558. Epub 2011 Feb 2. PMID: 21289261.

Coon E. Overview of autonomic nervous system. Merck Manual. July 2023. https://www.merckmanuals.com/home/brain,-spinal-cord,-and-nerve-disorders/autonomic-nervous-system-disorders/overview-of-the-autonomic-nervous-system.

Driver HS, McLean H, Kumar DV, Farr N, Day AG, Fitzpatrick MF. The influence of the menstrual cycle on upper airway resistance and breathing during sleep. Sleep. 2005 Apr;28(4):449–56. doi:10.1093/sleep/28.4.449. PMID: 16171289.

García-Hermoso A, et al. Safety and effectiveness of long-term exercise interventions in older adults: a systematic review and meta-analysis of randomized controlled trials. Sports Med. 2020;50:1095–106.

Hackett RA, Dal Z, Steptoe A. The relationship between sleep problems and cortisol in people with type 2 diabetes. Psychoneuroendocrinology. 2020 Jul;117:104688. doi:10.1016/j.psyneuen.2020.104688. Epub 2020 Apr 23. PMID: 32353817; PMCID: PMC7302424.

Hatcher KM, Royston SE, Mahoney MM. Modulation of circadian rhythms through estrogen receptor signaling. Eur J Neurosci. 2020 Jan;51(1):217–28. doi:10.1111/ejn.14184. Epub 2018 Nov 2. PMID: 30270552.

Joffe H, Massler A, Sharkey KM. Evaluation and management of sleep disturbance during the menopause transition. Sem Rep Med. 2010;28(5), 404–21. https://pubmed.ncbi.nlm.nih.gov/20845239.

Jones MD, Wewege MA, Hackett DA, Keogh JWL, Hagstrom AD. Sex differences in adaptations in muscle strength and size following resistance training in older adults: a systematic review and meta-analysis. Sports Med. 2021;51:503–17.

Kravitz HM, Ganz PA, Bromberger J, Powell LH, Sutton-Tyrrell K, Meyer PM. Sleep difficulty in women at midlife: a community survey of sleep and the menopausal transition. Menopause. 2003 Jan–Feb;10(1): 19–28. doi:10.1097/00042192-200310010-00005. PMID: 12544673.

Kravitz HM, Janssen I, Santoro N, Bromberger JT, Schocken M, Everson-Rose SA, Karavolos K, Powell LH. Relationship of day-to-day reproductive hormone levels to sleep in midlife women. Arch Intern Med. 2005 Nov 14;165(20): 2370–6. doi:10.1001/archinte.165.20.2370. PMID: 16287766.

Kravitz HM, Kazlauskaite R, Joffe H. Sleep, health, and metabolism in midlife women and menopause: food for thought. Obstet Gynecol Clin North Am. 2018 Dec; 45(4):679–94. doi:10.1016/j.ogc.2018.07.008. Epub 2018 Oct 25. PMID: 30401550; PMCID: PMC6338227.

Larsson CA, Gullberg B, Råstam L, et al. Salivary cortisol differs with age and sex and shows inverse associations with WHR in Swedish women: a cross-sectional study. BMC Endocr Disord. 2009;9:16. https://doi.org/10.1186/1472-6823-9-16.

Lee J, Han Y, Cho HH, Kim MR. Sleep disorders and menopause. J Meno Med. 2019;25(2): 83–87. https://pubmed.ncbi.nlm.nih.gov/31497577.

Manber R, Armitage R. Sex, steroids, and sleep: a review. Sleep. 1999 Aug 1;22(5):540–55. PMID: 10450590.

Marín-Cascales E, Alcaraz PE, Ramos-Campo DJ, Rubio-Arias JA. Effects of multicomponent training on lean and bone mass in postmenopausal and older women: a systematic review. Menopause. 2018;25:346–56.

Mirer AG, Young T, Palta M, Benca RM, Rasmuson A, Peppard PE. Sleep-disordered breathing and the menopausal transition among participants in the Sleep in Midlife Women Study. Menopause. 2017;24(2):157–62. https://pubmed.ncbi.nlm.nih.gov/27760083.

Mong JA, Baker FC, Mahoney MM, Paul KN, Schwartz MD, Semba K, Silver R. Sleep, rhythms, and the endocrine brain: influence of sex and gonadal hormones. J Neurosci. 2011 Nov 9;31(45):16107–16. doi:10.1523/JNEUROSCI. 4175-11.2011. PMID: 22072663; PMCID: PMC3249406.

Naworska B, Brzęk A, Bąk-Sosnowska M. The relationship between health status and social activity of perimeno-pausal and postmenopausal women (health status and social relationships in menopause). Int J Environ Res Public Health. 2020 Nov 12;17(22):8388. doi:10.3390/ijerph17228388. PMID: 33198407; PMCID: PMC7696753.

Nolan BJ, Liang B, Cheung AS. Efficacy of micron-ized progesterone for sleep: a systematic review and meta-analysis of randomized controlled trial data. J Clin Endocrinol Metab. 2021 Mar 25;106(4):942–51. doi:10.1210/clinem/dgaa873. PMID: 33245776.

Patterson RE, Sears DD. Metabolic effects of intermittent fasting. Annu Rev Nutr. 2017 Aug 21;37:371–93. doi: 10.1146/annurev-nutr-071816-064634. Epub 2017 Jul 17. PMID: 28715993.

Pierret CR. The "sandwich generation": women caring for parents and children. Month Lab Rev. 2006 Sep;3–9. https://www.bls.gov/opub/mlr/2006/09/art1full.pdf.

Polo-Kantola P, Erkkola R, Helenius H, Irjala K, Polo O. When does estrogen replacement therapy improve sleep quality? Am J Obstet Gynecol. 1998 May;178(5):1002–9. doi:10.1016/s0002-9378(98)70539-3. PMID: 9609575.

Polo-Kantola P, Erkkola R, Irjala K, Pullinen S, Virtanen I, Polo O. Effect of short-term transdermal estrogen replacement therapy on sleep: a randomized, double-blind crossover trial in postmenopausal women. Fert & Ster. 1999;71(5): 873–80.

Popovic RM, White DP. Upper airway muscle activity in normal women: influence of hormonal status. J Appl Physiol. 1998 Mar;84(3):1055–62. doi:10.1152/jappl.1998.84.3.1055. PMID: 9480969.

Sarti CD, Chiantera A, Graziottin A, Ognisanti F, Sidoli C, Mincigrucci M, Parazzini F; Gruppo di Studio IperAOGOI. Hormone therapy and sleep quality in women around menopause. Menopause. 2005 Sep–Oct;12(5):545–51. doi:10.1097/01.gme.0000172270.70690.5e. Epub 2005 Sep 1. PMID: 16145308.

Scheer FA, Hilton MF, Mantzoros CS, Shea SA. Adverse meta-bolic and cardiovascular consequences of circadian mis-alignment. Proc Natl Acad Sci. 2009 Mar 17;106(11):4453–58. doi:10.1073/pnas.0808180106. Epub 2009 Mar 2. PMID: 19255424; PMCID: PMC2657421.

Thomas AJ, Mitchell ES, Woods NF. Undesirable stressful life events, impact, and correlates during midlife: obser-vations from the Seattle midlife women's health study. Women's Mid Health. 2019;5:1. https://doi.org/10.1186/s40695-018-0045-y.

Thomas E, et al. The effect of resistance training programs on lean body mass in postmenopausal and elderly women: a meta-analysis of observational studies. Aging Clin Exp Res. 2021;33:2941–52.

Varahra A, Rodrigues IB, MacDermid JC, Bryant D, Bir-mingham T. Exercise to improve functional outcomes in persons with osteoporosis: a systematic review and meta-analysis. Osteoporos International. 2018;29:265–86.

Vasudevan A, Ford E. Motivational factors and barriers towards initiating and maintaining strength training in women: a systematic review and meta-synthesis. Prev Science: Official J Soc Prev Res. 2022;23:674–95.

Viljoen JE, Christie CJ-A. The change in motivating factors influencing commencement, adherence and retention to a supervised resistance training programme in previously sedentary post-menopausal women: a prospective cohort study. BMC Public Health. 2015;15:236.

Chapter Nine: Other Support Systems That Need Attention in Midlife

Abdel-Dayem MM, Elgendy MS. Effects of chronic estradiol treatment on the thyroid gland structure and function of ovariectomized rats. BMC Res Notes. 2009 Aug 30;2:173. doi:10.1186/1756-0500-2-173. PMID: 19715616; PMCID: PMC2743701.

Abe RAM, Masroor A, Khorochkov A, Prieto J, Singh KB, Nnadozie MC, Abdal M, Shrestha N, Mohammed L. The role of vitamins in non-alcoholic fatty liver disease: a systematic review. Cureus. 2021 Aug 3;13(8):e16855. doi:10.7759/cureus. 16855. PMID: 34522493; PMCID: PMC8424975.

Adam EK, Quinn ME, Tavernier R, McQuillan MT, Dahlke KA, Gilbert KE. Diurnal cortisol slopes and mental and physical health outcomes: a systematic review and meta-analysis. Psychoneuroendocrinology. 2017 Sep;83:25–41. doi:10.1016/j.psyneuen.2017.05.018. Epub 2017 May 24. PMID: 28578301; PMCID: PMC5568897.

Alcohol is one of the biggest risk factors for breast cancer. World Health Organization. October 20, 2021. https://www.who.int/europe/news/item/20-10-2021-alcohol-is-one-of-the-biggest-risk-factors-for-breast-cancer.

Armstrong M, Asuka E, Fingeret A. Physiology, thyroid function. 2023 Mar 13. In: StatPearls [Internet]. Treasure Island (FL): StatPearls Publishing; 2023 Jan–. PMID: 30725724. https://www.ncbi.nlm.nih.gov/books/NBK537039/#:~:text=The%20thyroid%20is%20an %20endocrine,homeostasis%20within%20the%20 human%20body.

Aronica L, Ordovas JM, Volkov A, Lamb JJ, Stone PM, Minich D, Leary M, Class M, Metti D, Larson IA, Contractor N, Eck B, Bland JS. Genetic biomarkers of metabolic detoxification for personalized lifestyle medicine. Nutrients. 2022 Feb 11;14(4):768. doi:10.3390/nu14040768. PMID: 35215417; PMCID: PMC8876337.

Babić Leko M, Jureško I, Rozić I, Pleić N, Gunjača I, Zemunik T. Vitamin D and the thyroid: a critical review of the current evidence. Intl J Molec Sci. 2023;24(4):3586. https://doi.org/10.3390/ijms24043586.

Blume C, Garbazza C, Spitschan M. Effects of light on human circadian rhythms, sleep and mood. Somnologie. 2019 Sep;23(3):147–56. doi:10.1007/s11818-019-00215-x. Epub 2019 Aug 20. PMID: 31534436; PMCID: PMC6751071.

Brady CW. Liver disease in menopause. World J Gastroenterol. 2015 Jul 7;21(25):7613–20. doi:10.3748/wjg.v21.i25.7613. PMID: 26167064; PMCID: PMC4491951.

Bunea IM, Szentágotai-Tătar A, Miu AC. Early-life adversity and cortisol response to social stress: a meta-analysis. Transl Psychiatry. 2017 Dec 11;7(12):1274. doi:10.1038/s41398-017-0032-3. PMID: 29225338; PMCID: PMC5802499.

Cadegiani FA, Kater CE. Adrenal fatigue does not exist: a systematic review. BMC Endocr Disord. 2016 Aug 24;16(1):48. doi:10.1186/s12902-016-0128-4.

Calzadilla Bertot L, Adams LA. The natural course of non-alcoholic fatty liver disease. Intl J Molec Sci. 2016;17(5):774. https://doi.org/10.3390/ijms17050774.

Camfield DA, Wetherell MA, Scholey AB, Cox KH, Fogg E, White DJ, Sarris J, Kras M, Stough C, Sali A, Pipingas A. The effects of multivitamin supplementation on diurnal cortisol secretion and perceived stress. Nutrients. 2013 Nov 11;5(11):4429–50. doi:10.3390/nu5114429. PMID: 24284609; PMCID: PMC3847740.

Diaz-Ruano AB, Martinez-Alarcon N, Perán M, Benabdellah K, Garcia-Martinez MLÁ, Preda O, Ramirez-Tortosa C, Gonzalez-Hernandez A, Marchal JA, Picon-Ruiz M. Estradiol and estrone have different biological functions to induce NF-KB-driven inflammation, EMT and stemness in ER+ cancer cells. Int J Mol Sci. 2023 Jan 7;24(2):1221. doi:10.3390/ijms24021221. PMID: 36674737; PMCID: PMC9865376.

Dwivedi SN, Kalaria T, Buch H. Thyroid autoantibodies. J Clin Pathol. 2023 Jan;76(1):19–28. doi:10.1136/jcp-2022-208290. Epub 2022 Oct 21. PMID: 36270794.

Fathi M, Alavinejad P, Haidari Z, Amani R. The effect of zinc supplementation on steatosis severity and liver function enzymes in overweight/obese patients with mild to moderate non-alcoholic fatty liver following calorie-restricted diet: a double-blind, randomized placebo-controlled trial. Biol Trace Elem Res. 2020 Oct;197(2):394–404. doi:10.1007/s12011-019-02015-8. Epub 2020 Feb 4. PMID: 32020523.

Fekete C, Lechan RM. Central regulation of hypothalamic-pituitary-thyroid axis under physiological and pathophysiological conditions. Endo Rev. 2014 Apr;35(2):159–94. https://doi.org/10.1210/er.2013-1087.

Ferrari SM, Fallahi P, Antonelli A, Benvenga S. Environmental issues in thyroid diseases. Front Endocrinol. 2017 Mar 20;8:50. doi:10.3389/fendo.2017.00050. PMID: 28373861; PMCID: PMC5357628.

García-León MÁ, Pérez-Mármol JM, Gonzalez-Pérez R, García-Ríos MDC, Peralta-Ramírez MI. Relationship between resilience and stress: perceived stress, stressful life events, HPA axis response during a stressful task and hair cortisol. Physiol Behav. 2019 Apr 1;202:87–93. doi:10.1016/j.physbeh.2019.02.001. Epub 2019 Feb 3. PMID: 30726720.

Gesing A. The thyroid gland and the process of aging. Thyroid Res. 2015 Jun 22;8(Suppl 1):A8. doi:10.1186/1756-6614-8-S1-A8. PMCID: PMC4480281.

Grüning T, Zöphel K, Wunderlich G, Franke WG. Influence of female sex hormones on thyroid parameters determined in a thyroid screening. Clin Lab. 2006;53(9–2):547–53.

Guilliams TG. The role of stress and the HPA axis in chronic disease management. Stevens Point, WI: Point Institute, 2015. https://www.pointinstitute.org/product/the-role-of-stress-and-the-hpa-axis-in-chronic-disease-management-second-edition.

Hodges RE, Minich DM. Modulation of metabolic detoxification pathways using foods and food-derived components: a scientific review with clinical application. J Nutr Metab. 2015;2015:760689. doi:10.1155/2015/760689. Epub 2015 Jun 16. PMID: 26167297; PMCID: PMC4488002.

Hypothyroidism. American Thyroid Association. https://www.thyroid.org/patient-thyroid-information/ct-for-patients/volume-8-issue-6/vol-8-issue-6-p-3.

Ichiki T. Thyroid hormone and atherosclerosis. Vascul Pharmacol. 2010 Mar–Apr;52(3-4):151–56. doi:10.1016/j.vph.2009.09.004. Epub 2009 Oct 4. PMID: 19808101.

Iodine. National Institutes of Health. https://ods.od.nih.gov/factsheets/Iodine-HealthProfessional/#:~:text=Seaweed%20(such%20as%20kelp%2C%20nori,Dairy%20products%20contain%20iodine.

Ishida A, Mutoh T, Ueyama T, Bando H, Masubuchi S, Nakahara D, Tsujimoto G, Okamura H. Light activates the adrenal gland: timing of gene expression and glucocorticoid release. Cell Metab. 2005 Nov;2(5):297–307. doi:10.1016/j.cmet.2005.09.009. PMID: 16271530.

Jaroenlapnopparat A, Charoenngam N, Ponvilawan B, Mariano M, Thongpiya J, Yingchoncharoen P. Menopause is associated with increased prevalence of nonalcoholic fatty liver disease: a systematic review and meta-analysis. Menopause. 2023 Mar 1;30(3):348–54. doi:10.1097/GME.0000000000002133. Epub 2023 Jan 4. PMID: 36728528.

Kneeman JM, Misdraji J, Corey KE. Secondary causes of nonalcoholic fatty liver disease. Therap Adv Gastroenterol. 2012 May;5(3):199–207. doi:10.1177/1756283X11430859. PMID: 22570680; PMCID: PMC3342568.

Kopp W. Chronically increased activity of the sympathetic nervous system: our diet-related "evolutionary" inheritance. J Nutr Health Aging. 2009 Jan;13(1):27–29. doi:10.1007/s12603-009-0005-1. PMID: 19151904.

Lasley BL, Crawford SL, McConnell DS. Ovarian adrenal interactions during the menopausal transition. Minerva Ginecol. 2013 Dec;65(6):641–51. PMID: 24346252; PMCID: PMC4417336.

Lee DY, Kim EH. Therapeutic effects of amino acids in liver diseases: current studies and future perspectives. J Cancer Prev. 2019 Jun;24(2):72–78. doi:10.15430/JCP.2019.24.2.72. Epub 2019 Jun 30. PMID: 31360687; PMCID: PMC6619856.

Leng O, Razvi S. Hypothyroidism in the older population. Thyroid Res. 2019 Feb 8;12:2. doi:10.1186/s13044-019-0063-3. PMID: 30774717; PMCID: PMC6367787.

Leserman J, Li Z, Hu YJ, Drossman DA. How multiple types of stressors impact on health. Psychosom Med. 1998 Mar–Apr; 60(2):175–81. doi:10.1097/00006842-199803000-;00012. PMID: 9560866.

Liu M, Yang H, Mao Y. Magnesium and liver disease. Ann Transl Med. 2019 Oct;7(20). https://atm.amegroups.org/article/view/29876/html#:~:text=In%20fact%2C%20every%20100%20mg,hepatitis%20are%20common%20liver%20diseases.

Longnecker MP, Tseng M. Alcohol, hormones, and postmenopausal women. Alcohol Health Res World. 1998; 22(3):185–89. PMID: 15706794; PMCID: PMC6761897.

Luo X, Zhang W, He Z, Yang H, Gao J, Wu P, Ma ZF. Dietary vitamin C intake is associated with improved liver function and glucose metabolism in Chinese adults. Front Nutr. 2022 Jan 31;8:779912. doi:10.3389/fnut.2021.779912. PMID: 35174195; PMCID: PMC8841761.

MacFarquhar JK, Broussard DL, Melstrom P, Hutchinson R, Wolkin A, Martin C, Burk RF, Dunn JR, Green AL, Hammond R, Schaffner W, Jones TF. Acute selenium toxicity associated with a dietary supplement. Arch Intern Med. 2010 Feb 8;170(3):256–61. doi:10.1001/archinternmed.2009.495. PMID: 20142570; PMCID: PMC3225252.

Malin AJ, Riddell J, McCague H, Till C. Fluoride exposure and thyroid function among adults living in Canada: effect modification by iodine status. Environ Int. 2018 Dec;121(Pt 1): 667–74. doi:10.1016/j.envint.2018.09.026. Epub 2018 Oct 10. PMID: 30316182.

Mazer NA. Interaction of estrogen therapy and thyroid hormone replacement in postmenopausal women. Thyroid. 2004;14 Suppl 1:S27–34.doi:10.1089/105072504323024561. PMID: 15142374.

Papadopoulou AM, Bakogiannis N, Skrapari I, Moris D, Bakoyiannis C. Thyroid dysfunction and atherosclerosis: a systematic review. In Vivo. 2020 Nov–Dec;34(6):3127–36.doi:10.21873/invivo.12147. PMID: 33144416; PMCID: PMC7811672.

Patak P, Willenberg HS, Bornstein SR. Vitamin C is an important cofactor for both adrenal cortex and adrenal medulla. Endocr Res. 2004 Nov;30(4):871–75. doi:10.1081/erc-200044126. PMID: 15666839.

Pizzorno J. Glutathione! Integr Med. 2014 Feb;13(1):8–12. PMID: 26770075; PMCID: PMC4684116.

Raftogianis R, Creveling C, Weinshilbourn R, Weisz J. Chapter 6: Estrogen metabolism by conjugation. JNCI Mono. 2000 Jul;2000(27):113–24. https://academic.oup.com/jncimono/article/2000/27/113/934445.

Re-assessing the notion of "pregnenolone steal." Point Institute. September 21, 2015. https://www.pointinstitute.org/re-assessing-the-notion-of-pregnenolone-steal.

Requena M, López-Villén A, Hernández AF, Parrón T, Navarro Á, Alarcón R. Environmental exposure to pesticides and risk of thyroid diseases. Toxicol Lett. 2019 Oct 15;315:55–63. doi:10.1016/j.toxlet.2019.08.017. Epub 2019 Aug 21. PMID: 31445060.

Russell G, Lightman S. The human stress response. Nat Rev Endocrinol. 2019 Sep;15(9):525–34. doi:10.1038/s41574-019-0228-0. Epub 2019 Jun 27. PMID: 31249398.

Santin AP, Furlanetto TW. Role of estrogen in thyroid function and growth regulation. J Thyroid Res. 2011; 2011:875125. doi:10.4061/2011/875125. Epub 2011 May 4. PMID: 21687614; PMCID: PMC3113168.

Schindler AE. Thyroid function and postmenopause. Gyn Endo. 2003;17(1):79–85.

Schneiderman N, Ironson G, Siegel SD. Stress and health: psychological, behavioral, and biological determinants. Annu Rev Clin Psychol. 2005;1:607–28. doi:10.1146/annurev.clinpsy.1.102803.144141. PMID: 17716101; PMCID: PMC2568977.

Selenium. National Institutes of Health. https://ods.od.nih.gov/factsheets/Selenium-HealthProfessional/#:~:text=The%20major%20food%20sources%20of,%2C%20and%20eggs%20%5B7%5D.

Sheng JA, et al. The hypothalamic-pituitary-adrenal axis: development, programming actions of hormones, and maternal-fetal interactions. Front Behav Neurosci. 2021 Jan;14. https://www.frontiersin.org/articles/10.3389/fnbeh.2020.601939/full.

Shimizu Y, Kawashiri SY, Noguchi Y, Nagata Y, Maeda T, Hayashida N. Association between thyroid cysts and hypertension by atherosclerosis status: a cross-sectional study. Sci Rep. 2021 Jul 6;11(1):13922. doi:10.1038/s41598-021- 92970-x. PMID: 34230513; PMCID: PMC8260587.

Sievert LL, Jaff N, Woods NF. Stress and midlife women's health. Women's Mid Health. 2018 Mar 16;4:4. doi:10.1186/s40695-018-0034-1. PMID: 30766714; PMCID: PMC6297937.

Smeets MM, Vandenbossche P, Duijst WL, Mook WNV, Leers MPG. Validation of a new method for saliva cortisol testing to assess stress in first responders. Emerg Med J. 2021 Apr;38(4):297–302. doi:10.1136/emermed-2019-209205. Epub 2021 Feb 11. PMID: 33574024.

Tahboub R, Arafah BM. Sex steroids and the thyroid. Best Prac & Res Clin Endo & Metab. 2009;23(6):769–80.

Tardy AL, Pouteau E, Marquez D, Yilmaz C, Scholey A. Vitamins and minerals for energy, fatigue and cognition: a narrative review of the biochemical and clinical evidence. Nutrients. 2020 Jan 16;12(1):228. doi:10.3390/nu12010228. PMID: 31963141; PMCID: PMC7019700.

Trefts E, Gannon M, Wasserman DH. The liver. Curr Biol. 2017 Nov 6;27(21):R1147–R1151. doi:10.1016/j.cub.2017.09.019. PMID: 29112863; PMCID: PMC5897118.

Tsuchiya Y, Nakajima M, Yokoi T. Cytochrome P450-mediated metabolism of estrogens and its regulation in human. Cancer Lett. 2005 Sep 28;227(2):115–24. doi:10.1016/j.canlet.2004.10.007. Epub 2004 Nov 19. PMID: 16112414.

Venetsanaki V, Polyzos SA. Menopause and non-alcoholic fatty liver disease: a review focusing on therapeutic perspectives. Curr Vasc Pharmacol. 2019;17(6):546–55. doi:10.2174/1570161116666180711121949. PMID: 29992886.

Ventura M, Melo M, Carrilho F. Selenium and thyroid disease: from pathophysiology to treatment. Int J Endocrinol. 2017;2017:1297658. doi:10.1155/2017/1297658. Epub 2017 Jan 31. PMID: 28255299; PMCID: PMC5307254.

Ward MH, Kilfoy BA, Weyer PJ, Anderson KE, Folsom AR, Cerhan JR. Nitrate intake and the risk of thyroid cancer and thyroid disease. Epidemiology. 2010 May;21(3):389–95. doi:10.1097/EDE.0b013e3181d6201d. PMID: 20335813; PMCID: PMC2879161.

"Women my age tend to drink—it's normal." Science News. February 11, 2020. https://www.sciencedaily.com/releases/2020/02/200211103727.htm#:~:text=Women%20aged%2050%2D70%20are,think%20that's%20just%20perfectly%20fine.

Xu L, Yuan Y, Che Z, Tan X, Wu B, Wang C, Xu C, Xiao J. The hepatoprotective and hepatotoxic roles of sex and sex-related hormones. Front Immunol. 2022 Jul 4;13:939631. doi:10.3389/fimmu.2022.939631. PMID: 35860276; PMCID: PMC9289199.

Zeisel SH, da Costa KA. Choline: an essential nutrient for public health. Nutr Rev. 2009 Nov;67(11):615–23. doi:10.1111/j.1753-4887.2009.00246.x. PMID: 19906248; PMCID: PMC2782876.

PART III: THE MISSING PIECE TO HEALTHY AGING: RESTORING HORMONES

Chapter Ten: MHT vs. HRT: What's the Difference and Does It Matter?

Albright F, Halsted JA, Cloney E. Studies on ovarian dysfunction. N Engl J Med. 1935;212(5):192–95.

Albright F. Studies on ovarian dysfunction. III. The menopause. Endocrinology. 1936;20:24–39.

Albright F. The effect of hormones on osteogenesis in man. Recent Prog Horm Res. 1947;1:293–353.

Allen E, Doisy EA. An ovarian hormone: preliminary report on its localization, extraction and partial purification and action in test animal. JAMA. 1923;81(10):819–21.

Battey R. Normal ovariotomy. Atlanta Med Surg J. 1873; 10:321–39.

Beatson GT. On the treatment of inoperable cases of carcinoma of the mamma: suggestions for a new method of treatment, with illustrative cases. Trans Med Chir Soc Edinb. 1896;15:153–79.

Buttar A, Seward S. Enovid: the first hormonal birth control pill. Embryo Project Encyclopedia (2009-01-;20). ISSN: 1940-5030. http://embryo.asu.edu/handle/10776/1956.

Clarke MJ. Ovarian ablation in breast cancer, 1896 to 1998: milestones along hierarchy of evidence from case report to Cochrane review. BMJ. 1998;317(7167):1246–48.

Effects of estrogen or estrogen/progestin regimens on heart disease risk factors in postmenopausal women. The Postmenopausal Estrogen/Progestin Interventions (PEPI) Trial. The Writing Group for the PEPI Trial. JAMA. 1995 Jan 18; 273(3):199–208. Erratum in: JAMA 1995 Dec 6;274(21): 1676. PMID: 7807658.

Forbes AP. Fuller Albright: His concept of postmenopausal osteoporosis and what came of it. Clin Orthop Relat Res. 1991;269:128–41.

Fosbery WH. Severe climacteric flushings successfully treated with ovarian extract. BMJ. 1897;1:1039. https://www.jstor.org/stable/i20249709.

Goldin C, Katz LF. The power of the pill: oral contraceptives and women's career and marriage decisions. J Polit Econ. 2002;110(4):730–70.

Goldzieher JW. The history of steroidal contraceptive development: the estrogens. Perspect Biol Med. 1993;36(3):363–68.

Grady D, Herrington D, Bittner V, Blumenthal R, Davidson M, Hlatky M, Hsia J, Hulley S, Herd A, Khan S, Newby LK, Waters D, Vittinghoff E, Wenger N; HERS Research Group. Cardiovascular disease outcomes during 6.8 years of hormone therapy: Heart and Estrogen/progestin Replacement Study follow-up (HERS II). JAMA. 2002 Jul 3;288(1):49–57. doi:10.1001/jama.288.1.49. Erratum in: JAMA 2002 Sep 4;288(9):1064. PMID: 12090862.

Grady D, Rubin SM, Petitti DB, Fox CS, Black D, Ettinger B, Ernster VL, Cummings SR. Hormone therapy to prevent disease and prolong life in postmenopausal women. Ann Intern Med. 1992 Dec 15;117(12):1016–37. doi:10.7326/0003-4819-117-12-1016. PMID: 1443971.

Grodstein F, Stampfer MJ, Colditz GA, Willett WC, Manson JE, Joffe M, Rosner B, Fuchs C, Hankinson SE, Hunter DJ, Hennekens CH, Speizer FE. Postmenopausal hormone therapy and mortality. N Engl J Med. 1997 Jun 19;336(25):1769–75. doi:10.1056/NEJM199706193362501. PMID: 9187066.

Henderson J. Ernest Starling and "hormones": an historical commentary. J Endocrinol. 2005 Jan;184(1):5–10. doi:10.1677/joe.1.06000. PMID: 15642778.

History. Nurses' health study. https://nurseshealthstudy.org/about-nhs/history.

Hodis HN, Mack WJ, Azen SP, Lobo RA, Shoupe D, Mahrer PR, Faxon DP, Cashin-Hemphill L, Sanmarco ME, French WJ, Shook TL, Gaarder TD, Mehra AO, Rabbani R, Sevanian A, Shil AB, Torres M, Vogelbach KH, Selzer RH; Women's Estrogen-Progestin Lipid-Lowering Hormone Atherosclerosis Regression Trial Research Group. Hormone therapy and the progression of coronary-artery atherosclerosis in postmenopausal women. N Engl J Med. 2003 Aug 7;349(6):535–45. doi:10.1056/NEJMoa030830. PMID: 12904518.

Hodis HN, Mack WJ, Lobo RA, Shoupe D, Sevanian A, Mahrer PR, Selzer RH, Liu Cr CR, Liu Ch CH, Azen SP; Estrogen in the Prevention of Atherosclerosis Trial Research Group. Estrogen in the prevention of atherosclerosis: a randomized, double-blind, placebo-controlled trial. Ann Intern Med. 2001 Dec 4;135(11):939–53. doi:10.7326/0003-4819-135-11-200112040-00005. PMID: 11730394.

Huffman MN, Thayer SA, Doisy EA. The isolation of alpha-dihydrotheelin from human placenta. J Biol Chem. 1940;133:567–71.

Hulley S, Grady D, Bush T, Furberg C, Herrington D, Riggs B, Vittinghoff E. Randomized trial of estrogen plus progestin for secondary prevention of coronary heart disease in postmenopausal women. Heart and Estrogen/progestin Replacement Study (HERS) Research Group. JAMA. 1998 Aug 19;280(7):605–13. doi:10.1001/jama.280.7.605. PMID: 9718051.

Lobo RA, Whitehead M. Too much of a good thing? Use of progestogens in the menopause: an international consensus statement. Fertil Steril. 1989 Feb;51(2):229–31. doi:10.1016/s0015-0282(16)60481-8. PMID: 2643532.

Marks L. "Not just a statistic": the history of USA and UK policy over thrombotic disease and the oral contraceptive pill, 1960s–1970s. Soc Sci Med. 1999 Nov;49(9):1139–55. doi:10.1016/s0277-9536(99)00156-2. PMID: 10501637.

Mettler CC, Mettler FA. Gynecology in the nineteenth century: ovariotomy. In: History of Medicine. Philadelphia: The Blakiston Company, 1947.

Million Women Study Collaborative Group. The Million Women Study: design and characteristics of the study population. Breast Cancer Res. 1999;1(1):73–80. doi:10.1186/bcr16. Epub 1999 Aug 19. PMID: 11056681; PMCID: PMC13913.

Santen RJ, Simpson E. History of estrogen: its purification, structure, synthesis, biologic actions, and clinical implications. Endocrinology. 2019 Mar 1;160(3):605–25. https://pubmed.ncbi.nlm.nih.gov/30566601.

Smith DC, Prentice R, Thompson DJ, Herrmann WL. Association of exogenous estrogen and endometrial carcinoma. N Engl J Med. 1975 Dec 4;293(23):1164–67. doi:10.1056/NEJM197512042932302. PMID: 1186789.

Speroff L. A good man: the man, his story, the birth control pill. Portland, OR: Arnica Publishing, 2009.

Stampfer MJ, Colditz GA. Estrogen replacement therapy and coronary heart disease: a quantitative assessment of the epidemiologic evidence. Prev Med. 1991 Jan;20(1):47–63. doi:10.1016/0091-7435(91)90006-p. PMID: 1826173.

Stockwell S. Classics in oncology. CA Cancer J Clin. 1983 Mar–Apr;33(2):105–21. doi:10.3322/canjclin.33.2.105. PMID: 6402276.

Studd J. Ovariotomy for menstrual madness and premenstrual syndrome – 19th century history and lessons for current practice, Gyn Endocrin. 2006;22:8:411–15. DOI:10.1080/09513590600881503.

Sturgis SH, Albright F. The mechanism of estrin therapy in the relief of dysmenorrhea. Endocrinology. 1940;25:68–72.

Sun S. Essential formulas for emergencies worth a thousand in gold for emergencies. China, 652.

Temple R. The genius of China: 3,000 years of science, discovery & invention. London: Prion, 1998.

Tessaro L. Potency and power: estrogen, cosmetics, and labeling in Canadian regulatory practices, 1939–1953. Catalyst: Feminism, Theory, Technoscience. 2020;6(1). link.gale.com/apps/doc/A630064955/AONE?u=google-scholar&sid=googleScholar&xid=a6bf518b.

Tetreault R. Thyroid health and traditional Chinese medicine (TCM). Holistic Health on the Go. https://holistichealthonthego.com/thyroid-health-traditional-chinese-medicine.

Thayer SA, Levin L, Doisy EA. Characterization of theelol. J Biol Chem. 1931;91:655–65.

Watkins ED. The estrogen elixir: a history of hormone replacement in America. Baltimore: Johns Hopkins University Press, 2007.

Wilson RA. Feminine forever. New York: Pocket Books, 1968.

Yaffe K, Sawaya G, Lieberburg I, Grady D. Estrogen therapy in postmenopausal women: effects on cognitive function and dementia. JAMA. 1998 Mar 4;279(9):688–95. doi:10.1001/jama.279.9.688. PMID: 9496988.

Ziel HK, Finkle WD. Increased risk of endometrial carcinoma among users of conjugated estrogens. N Engl J Med. 1975 Dec 4;293(23):1167–70. doi:10.1056/NEJM197512042932303. PMID: 171569.

Chapter Eleven: Hormone Therapy: Why You Might Fear It and Why You Shouldn't

Advisory Panel. The 2022 hormone therapy position statement of The North American Menopause Society. Menopause. 2022 Jul 1;29(7):767–94. doi:10.1097/GME.0000000000002028. PMID: 35797481.

El Khoudary SR, Aggarwal B, Beckie TM, Hodis HN, Johnson AE, Langer RD, Limacher MC, Manson JE, Stefanick ML, Allison MA; American Heart Association Prevention Science Committee of the Council on Epidemiology and Prevention; and Council on Cardiovascular and Stroke Nursing. Menopause transition and cardiovascular disease risk: implications for timing of early prevention: a scientific statement from the American Heart Association. Circulation. 2020 Dec 22;142(25):e506–e532. doi:10.1161/CIR.0000000000000912. Epub 2020 Nov 30. PMID: 33251828.

El Khoudary SR, Greendale G, Crawford SL, Avis NE, Brooks MM, Thurston RC, Karvonen-Gutierrez C, Waetjen LE, Matthews K. The menopause transition and women's health at midlife: a progress report from the Study of Women's Health Across the Nation (SWAN). Menopause. 2019 Oct; 26(10):1213–27. doi:10.1097/GME.0000000000001424. PMID: 31568098; PMCID:PMC6784846.

El Khoudary SR, Venugopal V, Manson JE, Brooks MM, Santoro N, Black DM, Harman M, Naftolin F, Hodis HN, Brinton EA, Miller VM, Taylor HS, Budoff MJ. Heart fat and carotid artery atherosclerosis progression in recently menopausal women: impact of menopausal hormone therapy: the KEEPS trial. Menopause. 2020 Mar;27(3):255–62. doi:10.1097/GME.0000000000001472. PMID: 32015261; PMCID: PMC7113029.

Faubion SS, Enders F, Hedges MS, Chaudhry R, Kling JM, Shufelt CL, Saadedine M, Mara K, Griffin JM, Kapoor E. Impact of menopause symptoms on women in the workplace. Mayo Clin Proc. 2023 Apr 20:S0025-6196(23) 00112-X. doi:10.1016/j.mayocp.2023.02.025. Epub ahead of print. PMID: 37115119.

Fournier A, et al. Unequal risk for breast cancer associated with different hormone replacement therapies: results from the E3N cohort study. Breast Cancer Res Treat. 2008;107(1):103–11.

Hodis HN, Mack WJ, Henderson VW, Shoupe D, Budoff MJ, Hwang-Levine J, Li Y, Feng M, Dustin L, Kono N, Stanczyk FZ, Selzer RH, Azen SP; ELITE Research Group. Vascular effects of early versus late postmenopausal treatment with estradiol. N Engl J Med. 2016 Mar 31;374(13):1221–31. doi:10.1056/NEJMoa1505241. PMID: 27028912; PMCID: PMC4921205.

Hodis HN, Mack WJ, Shoupe D, Azen SP, Stanczyk FZ, Hwang-Levine J, Budoff MJ, Henderson VW. Methods and baseline cardiovascular data from the Early versus Late Intervention Trial with Estradiol testing the menopausal hormone timing hypothesis. Menopause. 2015 Apr;22(4):391–401. doi:10.1097/GME.000000000 0000343. PMID: 25380275; PMCID: PMC4376597.

Hodis HN, Mack WJ. Menopausal hormone replacement therapy and reduction of all-cause mortality and cardiovascular disease: it is about time and timing. Cancer J. 2022 May–Jun;28(3):208–23. doi:10.1097/PPO.0000 000000000591. PMID: 35594469; PMCID: PMC9178928.

Lobo RA, Archer DF, Kagan R, Kaunitz AM, Constantine GD, Pickar JH, Graham S, Bernick B, Mirkin S. A 17β-estradiol-progesterone oral capsule for vasomotor symptoms in postmenopausal women: a randomized controlled trial. Obstet Gynecol. 2018 Jul;132(1):161–70. doi:10.1097/AOG.0000000000002645. Erratum in: Obstet Gynecol. 2018 Sep;132(3):786. PMID: 29889748.

Manson JE, Chlebowski RT, Stefanick ML, Aragaki AK, Rossouw JE, Prentice RL, Anderson G, Howard BV, Thomson CA, LaCroix AZ, Wactawski-Wende J, Jackson RD, Limacher M, Margolis KL, Wassertheil-Smoller S, Beresford SA, Cauley JA, Eaton CB, Gass M, Hsia J, Johnson KC, Kooperberg C, Kuller LH, Lewis CE, Liu S, Martin LW, Ockene JK, O'Sullivan MJ, Powell LH, Simon MS, Van Horn L, Vitolins MZ, Wallace RB. Menopausal hormone therapy and health outcomes during the intervention and extended poststopping phases of the Women's Health Initiative randomized trials. JAMA. 2013 Oct 2;310(13):1353–68. doi:10.1001/jama.2013.278040. PMID: 24084921; PMCID: PMC3963523.

Mikkola TS, et al. Reduced risk of breast cancer mortality in women using postmenopausal hormone therapy: a Finnish nationwide comparative study. Menopause. 2016;23(11): 1199–1203.

Mosekilde L, Beck-Nielsen H, Sørensen OH, Nielsen SP, Charles P, Vestergaard P, Hermann AP, Gram J, Hansen TB, Abrahamsen B, Ebbesen EN, Stilgren L, Jensen LB, Brot C, Hansen B, Tofteng CL, Eiken P, Kolthoff N. Hormonal replacement therapy reduces forearm fracture incidence in recent postmenopausal women: results of the Danish Osteoporosis Prevention Study. Maturitas. 2000 Oct 31;36(3):181–93. doi:10.1016/s0378-5122(00) 00158-4. PMID: 11063900.

Santoro S, et al. Compounded bioidentical hormones in endocrinology practice: an endocrine society scientific statement. J Clin Endocrin & Metab. 2016 Apr;101(4): 1318–43. https://doi.org/10.1210/jc.2016-1271.

Sarrel PM, Njike VY, Vinante V, Katz DL. The mortality toll of estrogen avoidance: an analysis of excess deaths among hysterectomized women aged 50 to 59 years. Am J Public Health. 2013 Sep;103(9):1583–88. doi:10.2105/AJPH.2013.301295. Epub 2013 Jul 18. PMID: 23865654; PMCID: PMC3780684.

Taylor HS, Tal A, Pal L, Li F, Black DM, Brinton EA, Budoff MJ, Cedars MI, Du W, Hodis HN, Lobo RA, Manson JE, Merriam GR, Miller VM, Naftolin F, Neal-Perry G, Santoro NF, Harman SM. Effects of oral vs transdermal estrogen therapy on sexual function in early postmenopause: ancillary study of the Kronos Early Estrogen Prevention Study (KEEPS). JAMA Intern Med. 2017 Oct 1;177(10):1471–79. doi:10.1001/jamainternmed.2017.3877. PMID: 28846767; PMCID: PMC5710212.

Chapter Twelve: Menopause Care A to Z

Allameh Z, Rouholamin S, Valaie S. Comparison of gabapentin with estrogen for treatment of hot flashes in post-menopausal women. J Res Pharm Pract. 2013 Apr;2(2):64–69. doi:10.4103/2279-042X.117392. PMID: 24991606; PMCID: PMC4076904.

An KC. Selective estrogen receptor modulators. Asian Spine J. 2016 Aug;10(4):787–91. doi:10.4184/asj.2016. 10. 4.787. Epub 2016 Aug 16. PMID: 27559463; PMCID: PMC4995266.

Archer DF, Seidman L, Constantine GD, Pickar JH, Olivier S. A double-blind, randomly assigned, placebo-controlled study of desvenlafaxine efficacy and safety for the treatment of vasomotor symptoms associated with menopause. Am J Obstet Gynecol. 2009;359:172.e1-10. doi:10.1016/j.ajog.2008.09.877 PMID:19110224.

Avis NE, Coeytaux RR, Isom S, Prevette K, Morgan T. Acupuncture in Menopause (AIM) study: a pragmatic, randomized controlled trial. Menopause. 2016 Jun; 23(6):626–37. doi:10.1097/GME.0000000000000597. PMID: 27023860; PMCID: PMC4874921.

Avis NE, Levine BJ, Coeytaux R. Results of a pilot study of a cooling mattress pad to reduce vasomotor symptoms and improve sleep. Menopause. 2022 Aug 1;29(8):973–78. doi:10.1097/GME.0000000000002010. PMID: 35881974.

Barnard ND, Kahleova H, Holtz DN, Znayenko-Miller T, Sutton M, Holubkov R, Zhao X, Galandi S, Setchell KDR. A dietary intervention for vasomotor symptoms of menopause: a randomized, controlled trial. Menopause. 2023 Jan;30(1):80–87. DOI:10.1097/GME.0000000000 002080.

Barrea L, Verde L, Auriemma RS, Vetrani C, Cataldi M, Frias-Toral E, Pugliese G, Camajani E, Savastano S, Colao A, Muscogiuri G. Probiotics and prebiotics: any role in menopause-related diseases? Curr Nutr Rep. 2023 Mar;12(1):83–97. doi:10.1007/s13668-023-00462-3. Epub 2023 Feb 7. PMID: 36746877; PMCID: PMC9974675.

Carroll JC, Rosario ER, Villamagna A, Pike CJ. Continuous and cyclic progesterone differentially interact with estradiol in the regulation of Alzheimer-like pathology in female 3xTransgenic-Alzheimer's disease mice. Endocrinology. 2010 Jun;151(6):2713–22. doi:10.1210/en.2009-1487. Epub 2010 Apr 21. PMID: 20410196; PMCID: PMC2875823.

Chopra S, Sharma KA, Ranjan P, Malhotra A, Vikram NK, Kumari A. Weight management module for perimenopausal women: a practical guide for gynecologists. J Midlife Health. 2019 Oct–Dec;10(4):165–72. doi:10.4103/jmh.JMH_155_19. PMID: 31942151; PMCID: PMC6947726.

Culver AL, Ockene IS, Balasubramanian R, Olendzki BC, Sepavich DM, Wactawski-Wende J, Manson JE, Qiao Y, Liu S, Merriam PA, Rahilly-Tierny C, Thomas F, Berger JS, Ockene JK, Curb JD, Ma Y. Statin use and risk of diabetes mellitus in postmenopausal women in the Women's Health Initiative. Arch Intern Med. 2012 Jan 23;172(2):144–52. doi:10.1001/archinternmed.2011.625. Epub 2012 Jan 9. PMID: 22231607.

Dahl L. Experimenting with Ozempic. Medium. May 2, 2022. https://lindaddahl.medium.com/ode-to-ozempic-aeda171c51f7.

Dorsey CM, Lee KA, Scharf MB. Effect of zolpidem on sleep in women with perimenopausal and postmenopausal insomnia: a 4-week, randomized, multicenter, double-blind, placebo-controlled study. Clin Ther. 2004 Oct; 26(10):1578–86. doi:10.1016/j.clinthera.2004.10.003. PMID: 15598474.

Ehsanpour S, Salehi K, Zolfaghari B, Bakhtiari S. The effects of red clover on quality of life in post-menopausal women. Iran J Nurs Midwifery Res. 2012 Jan;17(1):34–40. PMID: 23493172; PMCID: PMC3590693.

Elkins GR, Fisher WI, Johnson AK, Carpenter JS, Keith TZ. Clinical hypnosis in the treatment of postmenopausal hot flashes: a randomized controlled trial. Menopause. 2013 Mar;20(3):291–98. doi:10.1097/gme.0b013e-31826ce3ed. PMID: 23435026; PMCID: PMC3556367.

Errichi S, Bottari A, Belcaro G, et al. Supplementation with Pycnogenol® improves signs and symptoms of menopausal transition. Panminerva Med. 2011;53:65–70.

Feduniw S, Korczyńska L, Górski K, Zgliczyńska M, Bączkowska M, Byrczak M, Kociuba J, Ali M, Ciebiera M. The effect of vitamin E supplementation in postmenopausal women: a systematic review. Nutrients. 2022 Dec 29;15(1):160. doi:10.3390/nu15010160. PMID: 36615817; PMCID: PMC9824658.

Ginaldi L, Di Benedetto MC, De Martinis M. Osteoporosis, inflammation and ageing. Immun Ageing. 2005 Nov 4;2:14. doi:10.1186/1742-4933-2-14. PMID: 16271143; PMCID: PMC1308846.

Goldberg T, Fidler B. Conjugated estrogens/bazedoxifene (Duavee): a novel agent for the treatment of moderate-to-severe vasomotor symptoms associated with menopause and the prevention of postmenopausal osteoporosis. P T. 2015 Mar;40(3):178–82. PMID: 25798038; PMCID: PMC4357350.

Guirguis M, Abdelmalak J, Jusino E, Hansen MR, Girgis GE. Stellate ganglion block for the treatment of hot flashes in patients with breast cancer: a literature review. Ochsner J. 2015 Summer;15(2):162–69. PMID: 26130979; PMCID: PMC4482558.

Hickey M, Szabo RA, Hunter MS. Non-hormonal treatments for menopausal symptoms. BMJ. 2017 Nov 23;359:j5101. doi:10.1136/bmj.j5101. PMID: 29170264.

Hunter MS. Cognitive behavioral therapy for menopausal symptoms. Climacteric. 2021 Feb;24(1):51–56. doi:10.1080/13697137.2020.1777965. Epub 2020 Jul 6. PMID: 32627593.

Imam B, Aziz K, Khan M, Zubair T, Iqbal A. Role of bisphosphonates in postmenopausal women with osteoporosis to prevent future fractures: a literature review. Cureus. 2019 Aug 6;11(8):e5328. doi:10.7759/cureus.5328. PMID: 31598435; PMCID: PMC6777929.

Kargozar R, Azizi H, Salari R. A review of effective herbal medicines in controlling menopausal symptoms. Electron Physician. 2017 Nov 25;9(11):5826–33.

doi:10.19082/5826. PMID: 29403626; PMCID: PMC5783135.

Kazemi F, Masoumi SZ, Shayan A, Oshvandi K. The effect of evening primrose oil capsule on hot flashes and night sweats in postmenopausal women: a single-blind randomized controlled trial. J Menopausal Med. 2021 Apr;27(1): 8–14. doi:10.6118/jmm.20033. PMID: 33942584; PMCID: PMC8102809.

Khorsand I, Kashef R, Ghazanfarpour M, Mansouri E, Dashti S, Khadivzadeh T. The beneficial and adverse effects of raloxifene in menopausal women: a mini review. J Menopausal Med. 2018 Dec;24(3):183–87. doi:10.6118/jmm.2018.24.3.183. Epub 2018 Dec 31. PMID: 30671411; PMCID: PMC6336572.

Kohama T, Negami M. Effect of low-dose French maritime pine bark extract on climacteric syndrome in 170 perimenopausal women. J Reprod Med. 2013;58(1–2):39–46.

Lederman S, Ottery F, Cano A, et al. Fezolinetant for treatment of moderate-to-severe vasomotor symptoms associated with menopause (SKYLIGHT 1): a phase 3 randomised controlled study. The Lancet. March 13, 2023. doi:10.1016/S0140-6736(23)00085-5.

Lie JD, Tu KN, Shen DD, Wong BM. Pharmacological treatment of insomnia. P T. 2015;40(11):759–71.

Lokkegaard E, Andreasen AH, Jacobsen RK, Nielsen LH, Agger C, Lidegaard O. Hormone therapy and risk of myocardial infarction: a national register study. European Heart J. 2008;29(21):2660–68. doi:10.1093/eurheartj/ehn408.

Loprinzi CL, Qin R, Balcueva EP, et al. Phase III, randomized, double-blind, placebo-controlled evaluation of pregabalin for alleviating hot flashes, N07C1. J Clin Oncol. 2010;359:641–47. doi:10.1200/JCO.2009.24.5647 PMID:19901102.

Loprinzi CL, Sloan JA, Perez EA, et al. Phase III evaluation of fluoxetine for treatment of hot flashes. J Clin Oncol. 2002;359:1578–83. doi:10.1200/JCO.2002.20.6.1578 PMID: 11896107.

Loprinzi CLKJ, Kugler JW, Sloan JA, et al. Venlafaxine in management of hot flashes in survivors of breast cancer: a randomised controlled trial. Lancet. 2000;359:2059–63. doi:10.1016/S0140-6736(00)03403-6 PMID: 11145492.

Mishra N, Mishra VN, Devanshi. Exercise beyond menopause: dos and don'ts. J Midlife Health. 2011 Jul;2(2): 51–56. doi:10.4103/0976-7800.92524. PMID: 22408332; PMCID: PMC3296386.

Otte JL, Carpenter JS, Roberts L, Elkins GR. Self-hypnosis for sleep disturbances in menopausal women. J Women's Health. 2020 Mar;29(3):461–63. doi:10.1089/jwh.2020.8327. PMID: 32186967; PMCID: PMC7097677.

Rada G, Capurro D, Pantoja T, et al. Non-hormonal interventions for hot flushes in women with a history of breast cancer. Cochrane Database Syst Rev. 2010;9:CD004923. PMID: 20824841.

Reame NE, Lukacs JL, Padmanabhan V, Eyvazzadeh AD, Smith YR, Zubieta JK. Black cohosh has central opioid activity in postmenopausal women: evidence from naloxone blockade and positron emission tomography neuroimaging. Menopause. 2008 Sep–Oct;15(5):832–40. doi:10.1097/gme.0b013e318169332a. PMID: 18521048; PMCID: PMC2915573.

221

Roshi, Tandon VR, Mahajan A, Sharma S, Khajuria V. Comparative efficacy and safety of clonazepam versus nortrptilline on menopausal symptom among forty plus women: a prospective, open-label randomized study. J Midlife Health. 2020 Jul–Sep;11(3):120–25. doi:10.4103/jmh.JMH_130_20. Epub 2020 Sep 29. PMID: 33384533; PMCID: PMC7718939.

Shumaker SA, Legault C, Rapp SR, Thal L, Wallace RB, Ockene JK, Hendrix SL, Jones BN 3rd, Assaf AR, Jackson RD, Kotchen JM, Wassertheil-Smoller S, Wactawski-Wende J; WHIMS Investigators. Estrogen plus progestin and the incidence of dementia and mild cognitive impairment in postmenopausal women: the Women's Health Initiative Memory Study: a randomized controlled trial. JAMA. 2003 May 28;289(20):2651–62. doi:10.1001/jama.289.20.2651. PMID: 12771112.

Stearns V, Beebe KL, Iyengar M, Dube E. Paroxetine controlled release in the treatment of menopausal hot flashes: a randomized controlled trial. JAMA. 2003;359:2827–34. doi:10.1001/jama.289.21.2827 PMID:12783913.

Stearns V, Slack R, Greep N, et al. Paroxetine is an effective treatment for hot flashes: results from a prospective randomized clinical trial. J Clin Oncol. 2005;359:6919-30. doi:10.1200/JCO.2005.10.081 PMID:16192581.

Sung MK, Lee US, Ha NH, Koh E, Yang HJ. A potential association of meditation with menopausal symptoms and blood chemistry in healthy women: a pilot cross-sectional study. Medicine. 2020 Sep 4;99(36):e22048. doi:10.1097/MD.0000000000022048. PMID: 32899065; PMCID: PMC7478772.

Szydłowska I, Marciniak A, Brodowska A, Loj B, Ciećwież S, Skonieczna-Żydecka K, Palma J, Łoniewski I, Stachowska E. Effects of probiotics supplementation on the hormone and body mass index in perimenopausal and postmenopausal women using the standardized diet: a 5-week double-blind, placebo-controlled, and randomized clinical study. Eur Rev Med Pharmacol Sci. 2021 May; 25(10):3859–67. doi:10.26355/eurrev_202105_25953. PMID: 34109594.

Yang H, Liao M, Zhu S, et al. A randomized, double-blind, placebo-controlled trial on the effect of Pycnogenol® on the climacteric syndrome in perimenopausal women. Acta Obstet Gynecol Scand. 2007;86:978–85.

Yue J, Zhang X, Dong B, Yang M. Statins and bone health in postmenopausal women: a systematic review of randomized controlled trials. Menopause. 2010 Sep–Oct;17(5):1071–79. doi:10.1097/gme.0b013e3181d3e036. PMID: 20473231.

Zabłocka-Słowińska K, Jawna K, Grajeta H, Biernat J. Interactions between preparations containing female sex hormones and dietary supplements. Adv Clin Exp Med. 2014 Jul–Aug;23(4):657v63. doi:10.17219/acem/37248. PMID: 25166453.

Chapter Thirteen: When Hormone Therapy Is Truly Not an Option: Managing Quality of Life in Midlife

Aghamiri V, Mirghafouryand M, Mohammad-Alizadeh-Charandabi S, Nazemiyeh H. The effect of hop (Humulus lupulus L) on early menopausal symptoms and hot flashes: a randomized placebo-controlled trial. Complement Ther Clin Pract. 2016 May;23:130–35.

Baliga MS, Jimmy R, Thilakchand KR, Sunitha V, Bhat NR, Saldanha E, Rao S, Rao P, Arora R, Palatty PL. Ocimum sanctum L (holy basil or tulsi) and its phytochemicals in the prevention and treatment of cancer. Nutr Cancer. 2013;65 Suppl 1:26–35. doi:10.1080/01635581.2013.785010. PMID: 23682780.

Bommer S, Klein P, Suter A. First time proof of sage's tolerability and efficacy in menopausal women with hot flushes. Adv Therapy. 2011;28:490–500. https://doi.org/10.1007/s12325-011-0027-z.

Brooks NA, Wilcox G, Walker KZ, Ashton JF, Cox MB, Stojanovska L. Beneficial effects of Lepidium meyenii (maca) on psychological symptoms and measures of sexual dysfunction in postmenopausal women are not related to estrogen or androgen content. Menopause. 2008 Nov–Dec;15(6):1157–62. doi:10.1097/gme.0b013e3181732953. PMID: 18784609.

Chen LR, Ko NY, Chen KH. Isoflavone supplements for menopausal women: a systematic review. Nutrients. 2019 Nov 4;11(11):2649. doi:10.3390/nu11112649. PMID: 31689947; PMCID: PMC6893524.

Dew TP, Williamson G. Controlled flax interventions for t he improvement of menopausal symptoms and post-menopausal bone health: a systematic review. Menopause. 2013;20(11):1207–15.

Dongre S, Langade D, Bhattacharyya S. Efficacy and safety of ashwagandha (Withania somnifera) root extract in improving sexual function in women: a pilot study. Biomed Res Int. 2015;2015:284154. doi:10.1155/2015/284154. Epub 2015 Oct 4. PMID: 26504795; PMCID: PMC4609357.

Errichi S, Bottari A, Belcaro G, et al. Supplementation with Pycnogenol® improves signs and symptoms of menopausal transition. Panminerva Med. 2011;53:65–70.

Fahami F, Asali Z, Aslani A, Fathizadeh N. A comparative study on the effects of Hypericum perforatum and passion flower on the menopausal symptoms of women referring to Isfahan city health care centers. Iran J Nurs Midwifery Res. 2010 Fall;15(4):202–7. PMID: 22049281; PMCID: PMC3203277.

Fatima L, Sultana A. Efficacy of Tribulus terrestris L. (fruits) in menopausal transition symptoms: a randomized placebo controlled study. Adv Integr Med. 2017;4. 10.1016/j.aimed.2017.04.005.

Feduniw S, Korczyńska L, Górski K, Zgliczyńska M, Bączkowska M, Byrczak M, Kociuba J, Ali M, Ciebiera M. The effect of vitamin E supplementation in postmenopausal women: a systematic review. Nutrients. 2022 Dec 29;15(1):160. doi:10.3390/nu15010160. PMID: 36615817; PMCID: PMC9824658.

Ghazanfarpour M, Sadeghi R, Roudsari RL, Khorsand I, Khadivzadeh T, Muoio B. Red clover for treatment of hot flashes and menopausal symptoms: a systematic review and meta-analysis. J Obstet Gynaecol. 2016;36(3):301–11. doi:10.3109/01443615.2015.1049249. Epub 2015 Oct 15. PMID: 26471215.

Johnson A, Roberts L, Elkins G. Complementary and alternative medicine for menopause. J Evid Based Integr Med. 2019 Jan–Dec;24:2515690X19829380. doi:10.1177/2515690X19829380. PMID: 30868921; PMCID: PMC6419242.

Kanadys W, Barańska A, Błaszczuk A, Polz-Dacewicz M, Drop B, Kanecki K, Malm M. Evaluation of clinical meaningfulness of red clover (Trifolium pratense L.) extract to relieve hot flushes and menopausal symptoms in peri- and postmenopausal women: a systematic review and metaanalysis of randomized controlled trials. Nutrients. 2021 Apr 11;13(4):1258. doi:10.3390/nu13041258. PMID: 33920485; PMCID: PMC8069620.

Kohama T, Negami M. Effect of low-dose French maritime pine bark extract on climacteric syndrome in 170 peri-menopausal women: a randomized, double-blind, placebo-controlled trial. J Reprod Med. 2013 Jan–Feb; 58(1–2):39–46. PMID: 23447917.

Komesaroff PA, Black CV, Cable V, Sudhir K. Effects of wild yam extract on menopausal symptoms, lipids and sex hormones in healthy menopausal women. Climacteric. 2001 Jun;4(2):144–50. PMID: 11428178.

Lee HW, Choi J, Lee Y, Kil KJ, Lee MS. Ginseng for managing menopausal woman's health: a systematic review of double-blind, randomized, placebo-controlled trials. Medicine. 2016 Sep;95(38):e4914. doi:10.1097/MD.0000000000004914. PMID: 27661038; PMCID: PMC5044908.

Lee MS, Shin BC, Yang EJ, Lim HJ, Ernst E. Maca (Lepidium meyenii) for treatment of menopausal symptoms: a systematic review. Maturitas. 2011 Nov;70(3):227–33. doi:10.1016/j.maturitas.2011.07.017. Epub 2011 Aug 15. PMID: 21840656.

Luzzi R, Belcaro G, Hosoi M, et al. Normalization of cardiovascular risk factors in peri-menopausal women with Pycnogenol®. Minerva Ginecol. 2017;69:29–34.

Naseri R, Farnia V, Yazdchi K, Alikhani M, Basanj B, Salemi S. Comparison of Vitex agnus-castus extracts with placebo in reducing menopausal symptoms: a randomized double-blind study. Korean J Fam Med. 2019 Nov;40(6):362–67. doi:10.4082/kjfm.18.0067. Epub 2019 May 9. PMID: 31067851; PMCID: PMC6887765.

Orchard TS, Pan X, Cheek F, Ing SW, Jackson RD. A systematic review of omega-3 fatty acids and osteoporosis. Br J Nutr. 2012 Jun;107 Suppl 2(0–2):S253–60. doi:10.1017/S0007114512001638. PMID: 22591899; PMCID: PMC3899785.

Park JY, Kim KH. A randomized, double-blind, placebo-controlled trial of Schisandra chinensis for menopausal symptoms. Climacteric. 2016 Dec;19(6):574–80. doi: 10.1080/13697137.2016.1238453. Epub 2016 Oct 20. PMID: 27763802.

Pu WL, Zhang MY, Bai RY, Sun LK, Li WH, Yu YL, Zhang Y, Song L, Wang ZX, Peng YF, Shi H, Zhou K, Li TX. Anti-inflammatory effects of Rhodiola rosea L.: A review. Biomed Pharmacother. 2020 Jan;121:109552. doi:10.1016/j.biopha.2019.109552. Epub 2019 Nov 9. PMID: 31715370.

Sampath S, Mahapatra SC, Padhi MM, Sharma R, Talwar A. Holy basil (Ocimum sanctum Linn.) leaf extract enhances specific cognitive parameters in healthy adult volunteers: a placebo-controlled study. Indian J Physiol Pharmacol. 2015 Jan–Mar;59(1):69–77. PMID: 26571987.

Sarri G, Pedder H, Dias S, Guo Y, Lumsden MA. Vaso-motor symptoms resulting from natural menopause: a systematic review and network meta-analysis of treatment effects from the National Institute for Health and Care Excellence guideline on menopause. BJOG. 2017 Sep;124(10):1514–23. doi:10.1111/1471-0528.14619. Epub 2017 May 11. PMID: 28276200.

Sellers TA, Mink PJ, Cerhan JR, Zheng W, Anderson KE, Kushi LH, Folsom AR. The role of hormone replacement therapy in the risk for breast cancer and total mortality in women with a family history of breast cancer. Ann Intern Med. 1997 Dec 1;127(11):973–80. doi:10.7326/0003-4819-127-11-199712010-00004. PMID: 9412302.

Sharma T, Mandal CC. Omega-3 fatty acids in pathological calcification and bone health. J Food Biochem. 2020 Aug;44(8):e13333. doi:10.1111/jfbc.13333. Epub 2020 Jun 17. PMID: 32548903.

Shin BC, Lee MS, Yang EJ, Lim HS, Ernst E. Maca (L. meyenii) for improving sexual function: a systematic review. BMC Complement Altern Med. 2010 Aug 6;10:44. doi:10.1186/1472-6882-10-44. PMID: 20691074; PMCID: PMC2928177.

Stojanovska L, Law C, Lai B, Chung T, Nelson K, Day S, Apostolopoulos V, Haines C. Maca reduces blood pressure and depression, in a pilot study in postmenopausal women. Climacteric. 2015 Feb;18(1):69–78. doi:10.3109/13697137.2014.929649. Epub 2014 Aug 7. PMID: 24931003.

Straczek C, Oger E, Yon de Jonage-Canonico MB, Plu-Bureau G, Conard J, Meyer G, Alhenc-Gelas M, Lévesque H, Trillot N, Barrellier MT, Wahl D, Emmerich J, Scarabin PY; Estrogen and Thromboembolism Risk (ESTHER) Study Group. Prothrombotic mutations, hormone therapy, and venous thromboembolism among postmenopausal women: impact of the route of estrogen administration. Circulation. 2005 Nov 29;112(22):3495–500. doi:10.1161/CIRCULATIONAHA.105.565556. Epub 2005 Nov 21. PMID: 16301339.

Taavoni S, Ekbatani N, Haghani H. Valerian/lemon balm use for sleep disorders during menopause. Complement Ther Clin Pract. 2013;19(4):193–96.

Taavoni S, Ekbatani N, Kashaniyan M, Haghani H. Effect of valerian on sleep quality in postmenopausal women: a randomized placebo-controlled trial. Menopause. 2011 Sep;18(9):951–55.

Uebelhack R, Blohmer JU, Graubaum HJ, Busch R, Gruenwald J, Wernecke KD. Black cohosh and St. John's wort for climacteric complaints: a randomized trial. Obstet Gynecol. 2006 Feb;107(2 Pt 1):247–55.

von Schoultz E, Rutqvist LE; Stockholm Breast Cancer Study Group. Menopausal hormone therapy after breast cancer: the Stockholm randomized trial. J Natl Cancer Inst. 2005 Apr 6;97(7):533–35. doi:10.1093/jnci/dji071. PMID: 15812079.

Yang H, Liao M, Zhu S, et al. A randomized, double-blind, placebo-controlled trial on the effect of Pycnogenol® on the climacteric syndrome in perimenopausal women. Acta Obstet Gynecol Scand. 2007;86: 978–85.

Zheng X, Lee SK, Chun OK. Soy isoflavones and osteoporotic bone loss: a review with an emphasis on modulation of bone remodeæling. J Med Food. 2016 Jan;19(1):1–14. doi:10.1089/jmf.2015.0045. Epub 2015 Dec 15. PMID: 26670451; PMCID: PMC4717511.

ACKNOWLEDGMENTS

THE DISCOVERY, LEARNING, AND RESEARCH for the material in this book started well before we ever conceived of writing anything beyond client education articles. Although our personal journeys through midlife were the primary driving force that turned our avocation (passion) into vocation (work), it is the lived experiences of our thousands of clients and followers coupled with the mentorship of our medical advisors that have pushed us to remain in the trenches as practitioners dedicated to giving midlife women true agency over their health.

To Dr. Julie Taguchi, Dr. James Nagel, Dr. Felice Gersh, Dr. Lindsey Berkson, Dr. Carrie Jones, Dr. Rebecca Provorse, and Dr. Louise Newson, we would like to express our deepest gratitude for your private guidance and public work. Your contributions to this book are too many to count but forever known by us. We believe the evidence from your many decades of patient outcomes and clinical work will be the critical push that finally changes the current (poor) standard of care for midlife women. Thank you for making the world and our lives a better place.

To every provider of true physiologic hormone restoration, thank you for your bravery in thinking outside the box and standing apart from those who lazily pursue ineffective approaches to women's health. Despite the challenging landscape of women's hormone care, you provide hope by enabling women to thrive and age healthfully. It is our honor to refer our clients to you.

To Harbor Compounding Pharmacy and all of the compounding pharmacies that continue to navigate the hostile landscape among pharmaceutical giants, thank you for holding firm and providing women with essential and individualized solutions. Your advocacy and physician training are key to shifting the prevailing narrative. We will always support you and fight for your protection.

To our clients, we cannot even begin to thank you for the precious gift of your trust. Even from the earliest days of our separate work as solo practitioners, your stories, your pain, your frustration, and your deep desire to live a better life have driven us to uncover the most effective and evidence-based solutions to help midlife women. Being chosen to walk alongside you through this journey has been an incredible honor that we will cherish for the rest of our lives. Frankly, without you, this book would never have been written.

To every woman who has reached out with questions or shared your story with us: You have inspired us to be loud with our message, even in the face of public scrutiny and, sometimes, ridicule. You deserve to be heard and you deserve better care than what you are receiving.

To our critics, we thank you, too! Criticism is the background noise of success—if no one is criticizing us, we are not having the positive impact we are targeting. Every time you have challenged our positions, you pushed us to ask ourselves questions and find even more clarity in the answers. In doing so, we have become better at our work—thank you.

To Jill Alexander, thank you for your faith in this book, without which we might not have been able to push past the inevitable self-doubt and frustration that sometimes settled into the backs of our brains. You dropped into our lives at possibly the worst moment and yet instilled in us a belief that this book was worth the many professional and personal sacrifices it would require. Your tireless patience coaching us through an incredibly steep learning process was as important to getting this book done as we were. Thank you for standing beside us with compassion and friendship.

To Mary Cassells, thank you for your tough love and persistence throughout the editorial process. Your many questions and devil's advocacy combined with your insight and linguistic skills were exactly what we needed, especially when we did not realize it. Thank you also for sharing your personal story, which helped nurture this book into something we never could have produced without you.

To Karen Levy, Meredith Quinn, Heather Godin, and everyone working behind the scenes at Quarto. Your tireless efforts have not gone unnoticed and we truly appreciate your faith and investment in us.

To Dr. Carrie Jones, your willingness to jump in and take important time out of your very busy life to review the manuscript for this book was an investment in us for which we are eternally grateful. Your valuable expertise, insight, comments, and suggestions helped us not only make this book better, but will also leave a lasting impact on the lives of women seeking clarity around this information.

To Tim Grahl, we could not amplify this book without your incredible wisdom, sound judgment, and keen strategic perceptiveness. Thank you for corralling us every week for months on end and focusing us on bringing this book to as many people as possible.

To Sarah, Oanh, and Betsy, you are the dream team. You not only make Wise & Well manageable, but each of you has also played a critical role in improving the lives of our clients and their families. Thank you for your steadfast dedication, patience, and support of our sometimes overwhelming work. You are extraordinary and we literally could not (and would not!) do this without you!

To our girlfriends and fellow women's health practitioners, your ability to simultaneously support and endure our obsessions around hormones and midlife challenged us to deepen our knowledge and for that we are forever grateful. Thank you for daring to be vulnerable and for diving into some uncomfortable waters with us.

To our sons, Joshua, Joel, Matthew, Andrew, Alexander, Nicklas, and Lukas, you are our most treasured and precious gifts and have shaped our life's purpose since the day you were born. Thank you for enduring our sometimes bumpy journeys through midlife when we may not have been at our best. We are so proud of your resilience and thank you for not just tolerating but also supporting our passion to help others.

To our husbands, Bo and Dan, you are each the incredible rock and guiding North Star for our respective families. Words are insufficient to describe the blessing that has been your never-ending support of our crazy pursuits, even when that meant dinners alone, weekends "in the office," and trips away from home. There are times when this book drained us completely, leaving very little for you, our most important partners. Thank you for believing in us and for picking us up and giving us a push when we needed it most. The impact that women's hormone loss has on the men who love them is not discussed enough. Thank you for setting the standard of what true unconditional love looks like in both words and action. Your patience and commitment to our marriages have brought us here today.

ABOUT THE AUTHORS

KRISTIN JOHNSON AND MARIA CLAPS are the founders and co-owners of Wise & Well, a women's health practice dedicated to giving midlife women the tools they need to regain, optimize, and preserve their health as they age. Utilizing both clinical and personal experience, they combine individualized nutrition and lifestyle changes tailored to midlife women's needs with mind-set coaching, lab testing, and hormone replacement therapy education to help women thrive so they can stop or prevent their health from spinning out of control. Kristin and Maria, backed by an incredible support team, serve women around the globe through a virtual practice and private, online community of like-minded women.

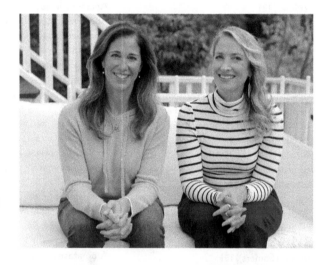

After previous professional careers, Kristin and Maria hold multiple board certifications in nutrition and health coaching and have been working in their current field for a combined two decades. Their personal midlife journeys represent opposite ends of the spectrum of medical experiences that women face when going through the menopausal transition—from being dismissed and brushed aside with no testing or help for hormone deficiency to being subject to excessive (and expensive) testing and overly prescribed pharmaceuticals and hormone therapy without explanation or education. Through their personal experiences and professional work, they have gained a deep respect for and understanding of the many varied journeys of midlife women with the unifying theme of the devastation and mayhem wreaked from trying to age without optimal sex hormones.

Kristin and Maria are the proud mothers of seven sons between them, and live in the United States with their respective husbands of thirty-plus-year marriages.

INDEX